Moving Beyond Prozac, DSM,
& the New Psychiatry

Corporealities: Discourses of Disability

David T. Mitchell and Sharon L. Snyder, editors

Moving Beyond Prozac, *DSM*, & the New Psychiatry

The Birth of Postpsychiatry

BRADLEY LEWIS

THE UNIVERSITY OF MICHIGAN PRESS   *Ann Arbor*

2009   2008   2007   2006   4   3   2   1

A CIP catalog record for this book is available from the British Library.

Library of Congress Cataloging-in-Publication Data

Lewis, Bradley, 1956–
    Moving beyond Prozac, DSM, and the new psychiatry : the birth of
postpsychiatry / Bradley Lewis.
        p. ; cm. — (Corporealities)
    Includes bibliographical references and index.
    ISBN-13: 978-0-472-11464-1 (cloth : alk. paper)
    ISBN-10: 0-472-11464-6 (cloth : alk. paper)
    ISBN-13: 978-0-472-03117-7 (pbk. : alk. paper)
    ISBN-10: 0-472-03117-1 (pbk. : alk. paper)
    1. Psychiatry—Methodology.   2. Psychiatry and the humanities.
3. Humanities.   I. Title.   II. Series.
    [DNLM: 1. Psychiatry.   2. Humanities.   3. Interdisciplinary
Communication.   4. Social Sciences.   WM 100 L673m 2006]
    RC437.5.L49 2006
    616.89—dc22   2005020756

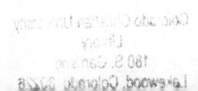

Acknowledgments

I am grateful to those many people who supported this book. Peter Caws, Stacy Wolf, and Mel Alexanderwitz provided the invaluable mentoring and support that enabled my early scholarship in the humanities. I am also greatly in debt to the kind and critical readership I received from Joanne Rendell, LeAnn Fields, Lennard Davis, Delese Wear, Marshall Alcorn, Gail Weiss, Barbara Miller, Jane Flax, James Griffin, Emily Martin, Suzanne Barnard, David DeGrazia, Andy Altman, Linda Morrison, Benny Rendell, Lisa Parker, Ken Thompson, Felice Aull, David Mitchell, Sharon Snyder, and Clair James. Finally, I would like to thank my colleagues and students over the years, most recently at New York University's Gallatin School of Individualized Study, for helping me work through and rehearse these many ideas.

I would also like to acknowledge the *Journal of Medical Humanities*, where earlier versions of chapters 5 and 7 were published.

Contents

Preface

For an array of historical and political reasons, contemporary psychiatry—what some call the "new psychiatry"—relentlessly champions science as its primary form of inquiry. This preference for science—the rhetoric of science, the methods of science, the company of scientists—cuts psychiatry off from the humanities, the arts, and the rest of intellectual thought. Psychiatry isolated from other human inquiries may map our brains or chart our neurotransmitters, but it becomes woefully inadequate for understanding our deepest human concerns. Narrowly specialized approaches to psychiatry have little hope of understanding the fullness of human desire, purpose, and suffering. And they have no hope of understanding the cultural contexts and political struggles that form the inescapable horizons of psychic life.

This book develops the theoretical tools and scholarly interchanges needed to address this imbalance. I write as a hybrid academic who trained in medicine and psychiatry before going back for a Ph.D. in the humanities and social theory. Here, employing recent theoretical work in the humanities to theorize contemporary psychiatry, I bring the two sides of my training together.

My goal in bringing the two sides of my training—in effect, the two sides of campus—together is to provide an alternative vision for psychiatry. Throughout this book, I employ the term *postpsychiatry* when referring to that alternative vision. The term was coined by two U.K. psychiatrists, Patrick Bracken and Philip Thomas, who like me are members of the Critical Psychiatry Network and part of an increasing chorus of people concerned with the reductionism of contemporary psychiatry.[1] Bracken and Thomas introduced the term to a wide audience in their *British Medical Journal* article "Postpsychiatry: A New Direction for Mental Health." In this article, they critique the modernist agenda in psychiatry and outline a "new positive direction for theory and practice in mental health" (2001, 724). They draw from recent theoretical work in the humanities to question modern psychiatry's Enlightenment legacy, particularly its preoccupations with science, universal truth, the individual subject, and one-sided notions of progress and advancement.

This vision of postpsychiatry does not reject or negate current psychiatry. Postpsychiatry is not a nostalgic return to psychoanalysis nor a radical antipsychiatry critique of mental illness as a myth. Rather, postpsychiatry moves the discussion forward by adding theoretical analysis of the many tensions within psychiatry and by opening psychiatry to alternative scholarly perspectives. That said, however, while postpsychiatry does not reject psychiatry, it does seriously shift the emphasis.

Contemporary psychiatry tends to focus on neurochemical and genetic explanations, to place technological solutions over ethical and human considerations, and to use forced treatment methods to resolve clinical controversy. Examples of these tendencies include the dramatic rise in psychopharmacologic (and poly-psychopharmacologic) treatment interventions, the rush toward DNA sequencing of psychic alienation and suffering, the growing reliance on diagnostic schedules and decision trees to sort out clinical ambiguities, and the increasing dependence on court mandates to force reluctant patients to "take their medications." By contrast, postpsychiatry works to counter these trends. As Bracken and Thomas put it, postpsychiatry "emphasizes social and cultural contexts, places ethics before technology, and works to minimize medical control of coercive interventions" (2001, 725).

Unfortunately, the reductionist trends in contemporary psychiatry will not change easily. In the last couple of decades, psychiatry's pendulum has swung so far toward a narrow scientific vision that much work needs to be done to develop a rich discourse in postpsychiatry. This book contributes to that effort by (1) working out a thick analysis of the theoretical materials needed for postpsychiatric thinking and critiques; (2) providing the scholarship necessary to build interdisciplinary alliances among psychiatry, the humanities, and social theory; and (3) developing strategies for creating critical interdisciplinary alternatives for psychiatric practice and knowledge creation.

The first chapter, "Theorizing Psychiatry," begins the process of linking psychiatry to contemporary humanities theory by exploring how the terms *theory* and *atheory* are used on the two sides of campus. Paradoxically, the term *theory* has diametrically opposite meanings in psychiatry and in the humanities. This chapter works through this contradiction and recommends that psychiatry adopt a perspective much more consistent with the humanities and social theory.

Inevitably, adopting this kind of theoretical perspective exposes postpsychiatry to recent debates in the "science wars." These debates, which center on the question of reality and whether science represents the real world or is itself socially constructed, have stirred heated controversy across campus. Chapter 2, "Dodging the Science Wars," outlines the battle lines between these realist and constructivist visions and argues for a third position based on a general theory of representation as applied to psychiatry.

Chapter 3, "The New Psychiatry as a Discursive Practice," focuses on the work of philosopher Michel Foucault and his theory of "discursive practice." Foucault is invaluable to postpsychiatry because, in addition to sidestepping the realist and constructionist traps, he adds the human "power" dimensions of representation. As Foucault showed, representational practices like the new psychiatry do not arise spontaneously; they emerge through a dense web of human relations and political power struggles.

Chapter 4 offers a sustained reflection on modernism and postmodernism as relevant to psychiatry. "Psychiatry and Postmodern Theory" outlines three themes of psychiatric modernism and contrasts these with three themes of psychiatric postmodernism—or postpsychiatry, bringing together much of the theoretical work in the earlier chapters and setting the stage for the more applied work in the later chapters.

Chapter 5, "Postdisciplinary Coalitions and Alignments," connects postpsychiatry to applied scholarly work in a lively new area: cultural studies of psychiatry, which can serve as an interdisciplinary home and useful model for postpsychiatry. Cultural studies approaches suggest ways that theoretical materials from the humanities can be applied to specific psychiatric issues and concerns, demonstrating how coalitions can be fruitfully built among the humanities, social theory, and psychiatry.

The next two chapters offer examples of such cultural studies of psychiatry, looking at two key phenomena in contemporary psychiatry. Chapter 6, "Decoding *DSM:* Bad Science, Bad Rhetoric, Bad Politics," focuses on the creation, during the 1970s and 1980s, of the "bible" of scientific psychiatry: the third edition of the *Diagnostic and Statistical Manual (DSM-III)*. This edition (and the many revisions that followed) allowed contemporary psychiatry to define itself as "theoretically neutral" and "scientific." Critical commentary on the manual has tended to focus on its very problematic scientific claims, but such analysis does not allow us to fully understand the manual. Why did the manual emerge when it did? What were the struggles and controversies surrounding it? How were they resolved? Who were the main players? What were their politics? There was much more involved in the manual's creation than just bad scientific judgments. All of the bad choices surrounding the manual (scientific, rhetorical, and political) were made by particular people with particular interests. This chapter brings to light who these people were, the choices they made, and how they interacted with each other.

Chapter 7, "Prozac and the Posthuman Politics of Cyborgs," moves to the 1990s—the period the first President George Bush called "The Decade of the Brain." There is a direct link between the publication of the *DSM-III* and advancement of the "new scientific psychiatry" and the obsessive interest in the brain that followed. A careful cultural analysis of the phenomenon of Prozac, the immensely popular prescription drug for depression, provides a particularly fruitful way to understand this period. Something remarkable happened in contemporary psychiatry when Prozac was introduced. This chapter explores the Prozac story and the brain frenzy that surrounded it.

Chapter 8, "Postempiricism: Imagining a Successor Science for Psychiatry," moves beyond analysis and critique to imagine an alternative future for psychiatric research and knowledge creation, using both Foucault and feminist postepistemology. The exploration here is more creative than it is politically feasible, attempting to freely imagine how things might be otherwise and to provide illumination that could inform and inspire potential reform efforts.

The epilogue, "Postpsychiatry Today," considers the possibilities for building a knowledge base in postpsychiatry without an ideally restructured successor science. The focus here is on two rapidly growing domains, disability studies and medical humanities, which have proven to be exemplary in their interdisciplinary and cross-campus scholarship and alliances. Both are sites in which postpsychiatric scholarship and cross-campus alliances could also flourish. The book concludes with suggestions for ways that both clinicians and consumers might begin shifting their work toward a postpsychiatry model.

Although this book is in many places critical of the field, I write as an advocate of psychiatry, both as a consumer and as a provider, who has had many rich and rewarding experiences with psychiatry. My own psychotherapy, which lasted for several years, has been the single best thing I ever did for myself. I am more thoughtful, more flexible, more capable, more loving, more joyful, and more at peace because of psychotherapy. And in my work as a practicing psychiatrist, I have been fortunate in assisting hundreds of people to make amazing changes in their lives—many of whom used psychiatry to enable them along the way.

I believe in psychiatry. I believe that secular cultures need the services psychiatry can provide. At its best, psychiatric care provides holding spaces where people may come for help with their confusions, their suffering, and their anxieties, without judgment or blame. Ideally, people in need should meet kind, thoughtful, and well-trained clinicians who are happy in their work. These clinicians should have a broad education and be aware of the multiple dimensions of human suffering and human flourishing. They should also have the generosity of spirit to help wherever they can and the humility and wisdom to recognize those instances where they can provide only companionship and solace.

To nurture that kind of clinician, psychiatry must reconsider its basic priorities, as that caliber of clinician requires scholarly resources beyond the sciences. Although an advocate for psychiatry, I am deeply worried about its soul and its future. I yearn for a psychiatry that lives up to its potential as a helping profession. Psychiatry's current path is taking it further and further from that potential. It is difficult these days to find well-rounded and intellectually nuanced psychiatrists. The best way to correct this imbalance toward science and rationality is to develop alliances on both sides of campus that will bring the tools and insights of the humanities to bear on the training of psychiatrists. This book is an effort to move in that direction.

CHAPTER ONE

Theorizing Psychiatry

The story of U.S. psychiatry in the latter half of the twentieth century is a story of transition and paradigm shift. Anthropologist T. M. Luhrmann makes this clear in her recent ethnography of psychiatry, *Of Two Minds*. At the end of World War II, she writes, "psychoanalysis completely dominated psychiatry and was nearly synonymous with [the field]" (2000, 212). Psychoanalysis provided the leading explanation for mental illness, and it provided the leading treatments. However, by the 1970s and 1980s, psychoanalytic dominance in psychiatry was over. Though there continue to be occasional struggles, for the most part biological psychiatry has successfully supplanted psychoanalysis in all of its former positions of leadership. These changes are not subtle. They do not merely fine-tune or "correct" psychoanalysis; they completely overthrow it. For biopsychiatry, not only is psychoanalysis over, but "psychoanalysis is charlatanry and psychiatric disorder is brain dysfunction" (Luhrmann 2000, 203). This new dominance of biological psychiatry brings with it many things. The most well-known is an increased emphasis on pharmaceutical treatments. But even more important, the new biological psychiatry brings with it an enhanced narrative of "scientific method" and an amazingly idealized notion of "theory neutrality."

On the other side of campus, equally dramatic changes have occurred in the humanities and parts of the social sciences. At the end of World War II, there was a consensus that the humanities rested on neutral distinctions between fact and value, theory and observation, and knowledge and power. Value neutrality and theory neutrality were hallmark principles of humanities scholars who, like their scientific colleagues, maintained an austere posture of objectivity. But as humanities observers M. Kreiswirth and M. Cheetham point out, the "theory wars of the 1970's and 1980's" changed all that. With the rise of theory, commonsense distinctions between fact and value, theory and observation, and knowledge and power were blurred beyond recognition. Though there continue to be skirmishes, there is little doubt that today theory has become a hallmark of contemporary humanities and the intellectual community at large. For the new theoretical humanities, "not only may we be 'theory-mad beyond redemption'—to borrow a phrase of Poe's—but we may even wonder how desirable such redemption might be, or indeed, how it might be possible to envision it without what we now call theory" (Kreiswirth and Cheetham 1990, 1).

Thus, over the last thirty years, a curious contradictory trend has occurred on the two sides of U.S. campuses. Clinical and research psychiatry has rallied itself with great fervor to champion "atheoretical" psychiatric knowledge, while, during that same period, the humanities have gone in the exact opposite direction to become "theory-mad beyond redemption." This chapter contemplates this contradiction by detailing the rise of psychiatry's "atheoretical" trope and considering the functions it serves in contemporary psychiatry. I use science studies literature to raise doubts about the necessity of psychiatry's atheoretical self-conception. Science studies suggests that atheoretical psychiatry is not inevitable and that it is only one option among many possibilities. There are many other ways to understand science than through the trope of "theory neutrality," and science studies scholarship provides some wiggle room to get out of the box of psychiatry's atheoretical approach.

Once outside the box, another option and potential real choice for psychiatry emerges: theorized postpsychiatry. The "theory" for this option does not come from nowhere. It comes from theoretical work in the humanities. But this humanities theory is complicated, composed of multiple interrelated strands with multiple ways it may be narrated (Leitch 2003). Thus, before going on to apply humanities theory to postpsychiatry, I will spend some time unpacking the question of what is theory in the humanities.

The Rise of Atheoretical Psychiatry

In 1980, when the American Psychiatric Association (APA) published a revised version of its standard diagnostic manual, the third edition of the *Diagnostic and Statistical Manual of Mental Disorders* (*DSM-III*), U.S. psychiatry underwent what many are calling a scientific revolution. These two events, the publishing of *DSM-III* and the concurrent rise in scientific psychiatry, also hailed the emergence of "atheoretical psychiatry." I put "atheoretical" in quotation marks as a way to bracket off the truth of psychiatry's atheoretical claim. I'm not exploring here whether psychiatry really is atheoretical. Rather, I'm interested in how psychiatry came to understand itself as atheoretical.

Gerald Maxmen's book *The New Psychiatry* is a good place to start. Maxmen congratulates psychiatry for its emerging scientific status and sums up nicely the effect of *DSM-III* on "scientific psychiatry" with the following proclamation:

> On July 1, 1980, the ascendance of scientific psychiatry became official. For on this day, the APA published a radically different system for psychiatric diagnosis called . . . *DSM-III*. By adopting the scientifically based *DSM-III* as its official system for diagnosis, American psychiatrists broke with a fifty-year tradition of using psychoanalytically based diagnoses. Perhaps more than any other single event, the publication of *DSM-III* demonstrated that American psychiatry had indeed undergone a revolution. (1985, 35)

In Maxmen's historical narrative, the rise of scientific psychiatry and the publication of *DSM-III* are part of the same pattern of changes, or the same "scientific revolution," through which psychiatry has passed over the last twenty years. Maxmen's narrative is a tale of Enlightenment progress. For Maxmen and the new psychiatry, more science equals more progress. The qualifier "more" is important, because it is not simply that the old "psychoanalytic" approaches were not scientific. Indeed, psychoanalysis itself rode on a narrative of scientific progress (Freud 1954). Freud was often at pains to point out that psychoanalysis was a "scientific psychology"—which in Freud's own Enlightenment narrative is why psychoanalysis was superior to philosophy or religion. But for Maxmen and the new psychiatry, psychoanalysis is not scientific enough. Indeed, for Maxmen, psychoanalysis is so close to religion and philosophy that it is only with the *DSM-III* that psychiatry truly achieves a scientific revolution.

Maxmen is not alone in marking the turning point toward a new scientific psychiatry with the publication of *DSM-III*. Though he is perhaps unique in his religio-secular fervor ("For on this day, the APA published a radically different system of psychiatric diagnosis"), other psychiatric commentators are in general agreement that *DSM-III* marks the beginning of the new scientific psychiatry. For example, Robert Spitzer, *DSM-III*'s principal architect, calls the manual a "signal achievement for psychiatry" and "an advance toward the fulfillment of the scientific aspirations of the profession" (Bayer and Spitzer 1985, 187). In chorus with Spitzer, acclaimed psychiatrist Gerald Klerman, speaking at the 1982 APA conference, asserts:

> *DSM-III* represents a fateful point in the history of the American psychiatric profession. . . . The decision of the APA first to develop *DSM-III* and then to promulgate its use represents a significant reaffirmation on the part of American psychiatry to its medical identity and its commitment to scientific medicine. (1984, 539)

In a similar vein, the latest edition of the APA manual, *DSM-IV,* uses an only a slightly more moderate tone to call *DSM-III* a "major advance" that has "greatly facilitated empirical research" (American Psychiatric Association 1994, xviii). Clearly the inauguration or, better yet, the coronation of *DSM-III* has been a turning point in the new psychiatry's self-understanding as a more rigorous science.

The new *DSM-III* brought not only a heightened scientific psychiatry but also an atheoretical or theoretically neutral psychiatry. Joseph Margolis argues, in a philosophical review of *DSM-III*, that theory neutrality is its "master theme" (1994, 106). Margolis does not have a difficult time making this argument. Indeed, the insight that theory neutrality is the master theme of *DSM-III* requires little philosophy. Spitzer makes the goal of theory neutrality plain both in his introduction to the *DSM-III* and again in a review of *DSM-III*'s method: "[*DSM-III*] takes an atheoretical approach with respect to etiology" (Margolis 1994, 106). Spitzer's justification is as follows:

> Given the present state of ignorance about etiology, we should avoid including etiological assumptions in the definitions of the various mental disorders, so that people with different theories about etiology can at least agree on the features of the various disorders without having to agree on how those disorders came about. (Margolis 1994, 106)

From this we see a core originating impulse of *DSM-III:* to be theory neutral with respect to etiology. This state of affairs has changed little in recent years. Though the *DSM-III*'s goal of "theory neutrality" has been extensively criticized (see Margolis for an example), the recent publication of the latest *DSM* reproduces this same theme. According to *DSM-IV*'s introduction, the uniqueness of *DSM-III* was that it formally introduced into psychiatry the "important methodological innovation" of a "descriptive approach [to psychiatric diagnosis] that attempts to be *neutral with respect to theories*" (American Psychiatric Association 1994, xviii, italics added). Margolis's conclusion that theory neutrality is the "master theme" of *DSM-III* clearly captures the rhetoric of the new *DSM-IV* as well.

This continuation of theory neutrality into *DSM-IV* is not particularly surprising, and it will be quite difficult for psychiatry to give up its new-found "atheoretical" identifications. According to the "scientific revolution" narrative of the new psychiatry, *DSM-III*'s theory neutrality finally allowed psychiatry to rid itself of prejudice and superstition and thus take its rightful place among the objective sciences. The new psychiatry sees the move to an atheoretical, scientific *DSM-III* as a move from psychiatric Myth to psychiatric Truth. This will not be an easy identity to shake. Richard Wyatt (former chief of the Adult Psychiatry Branch, Division of Intramural Research, National Institute of Mental Health, and an important contributor to the rise of scientific psychiatry) proudly puts it this way:

> Good psychiatry requires careful observations and descriptions, *unvarnished by theory*. This point is demonstrated by the changes made from the second edition of the *Diagnostic and Statistical Manual of Mental Disorders* (*DSM-II*) to the third edition (*DSM-III*); the latter is an attempt to describe things as they are, but the former often blurred observations and interpretations. *DSM-III* adds objectivity, reliability, and prognostic validity. . . . It uses the minimal level of inference necessary to characterize the disorder. This movement toward clear, unambiguous description of psychiatric syndromes lays an important foundation for correlative and experimental exploration of the psychiatric illnesses. (1985, 2018, italics added)

Wyatt interprets "good psychiatry" as psychiatry that operates with the benefits of *DSM-III*'s improved scientific methodology. Good psychiatry, for Wyatt, operates without the distortions of theory and progressively advances toward the "unambiguous description" of psychiatric syndromes and their eventual treatment. For Wyatt, the advance of science in psychiatry leads unquestionably toward advance in psychiatry. What is good for science in psychiatry is good for psychiatry.

As a consequence, "bad psychiatry," for Wyatt, can be understood as psychiatry that relies on what he calls "blurred" alternatives. In short, bad psychiatry is based on nonscientific, non-*DSM-III* approaches. The amazing result of this rhetoric is that any approaches to psychiatric problems not based on *DSM-III*—whether they be psychoanalytic, existential, family, social, political, philosophical, pastoral, narrative, or cultural—are simultaneously put out of play. These alternative approaches do not have to be addressed directly on their own merit or even tended to in their specifics. They are simply dismissed through an all-encompassing charge that, like superstition, they are little more than confused smears of "blurred observations and interpretations."

Science Studies and the Critiques of Atheoretical Science

Thus, the new psychiatry has come to organize itself around a trope of "atheoretical science." But is science best understood as atheoretical? Are there other ways to understand how science works? If so, what are the effects and consequences of alternative understandings? Questions like these are rarely posed in the literature on scientific psychiatry. One can find very little debate on the move toward theory neutrality within the new psychiatric literature, because the new psychiatry simply assumes that science is "atheoretical" and that it is the obvious route to "progress." These are the founding assumptions on which psychiatry has justified its revolution. However, when one steps outside the psychiatric literature to evaluate and analyze this assumption, there is a wealth of scholarly material that would suggest a much more complex perspective on science.

Science studies is the umbrella term that encompasses scholars who focus on the rules, norms, methods, expectations, and consequences of science. Anthropologist David Hess attempts to sort out and simplify the ever-proliferating arena of science studies by dividing it into four broad genres or research traditions: history and philosophy of science, sociology of science, social studies of scientific knowledge, and feminist and cultural studies of science. Hess argues that although science studies is not unanimous and is at times quite acrimonious, as a whole it provides a rich "conceptual tool kit" for a more nuanced and complex understanding of the very possibility of an "atheoretical" model for science, technology, or medicine (1997, 1).

What have science studies scholars come to understand about science? Science studies scholar Sharon Traweek articulates several widely accepted "findings" of the last thirty years of science studies research (1996, 140). Most of these findings are correctives to the "received view" of science as objective and theory neutral. For Traweek, the received view of science includes the following assumptions:

- The scientific method identifies and controls all variables in an experiment.
- Scientific knowledge is amassed progressively and cumulatively.
- Scientific reasoning proceeds by deduction and induction; hypotheses are deduced from existing experimental data, and experimental data are tested against hypotheses inductively.
- Scientific research is made objective by eliminating all biases and emotions of the researchers.
- Scientific research is neutral with respect to social, political, economic, ethical, and emotional concerns.
- Scientific research has an internal intellectual logic; there is [also] an external social, political, economic, and cultural context for science that can only affect which scientific ideas are funded or applied.
- Improvements in the quality of human life and the duration of human life during the past two hundred years are due primarily to the application of scientific discoveries.
- Technology is applied science.
- Basic research and applied research are easily differentiated.
- There is a significant rate of "social return" on scientific research.
  (From Traweek 1996, 141)

According to Traweek, these received views of science are usually narrated indirectly in the form of what she calls "reverential stories." These stories include a "list of saints' (geniuses') lives, their miracles (discoveries), and holy sites (laboratories) and can usually be found in television documentaries, basic textbooks, and official histories of science" (1996, 141). Because psychiatry has recently adopted this very same received view of science, it is perhaps not surprising that the new psychiatry is also rapidly putting together its own reverential story (like the one found in Maxmen's *The New Psychiatry*) centering around the recent miracle of *DSM-III* and the saints who devoted themselves to its development.

The received views of science, however, have been powerfully challenged by the last thirty years of science studies. From Traweek's perspective (though like Hess she finds science studies not to be a unified whole), science studies scholars generally agree on basic alternatives to the received view (1996, 148). These largely held agreements include the following:

- There are many practices called "science" by their practitioners, not one such practice; there are many methods called "scientific method" by their practitioners, not one such method. That is, each research subfield has its own distinctive research practices. Hence, the proper terms are plural: *sciences* and *scientific methods.*

- The forms used in scientific writing have converged and have not varied significantly over the last couple of centuries. For example, all references to the agency of the scientists involved in the research are minimized. The written presentation of findings has become quite stylized and terse; it would be almost impossible to reproduce an experiment based upon the information provided in scientific articles.

- Access to scientific knowledge is highly restricted. That is, there is restricted access to different stages of training and to findings, positions, publications, and conferences—the whole infrastructure of knowledge production and consumption.

- Problem selection is a process highly subject to the available resources.

- Adjudicating which experimental data to take as facts and which theories to take as important is a collective process conducted by those who are tacitly empowered with the authority to participate; it does not include all practicing scientists in a particular field.

- Closure of debates about the status of data and theories is not accomplished with definitive findings as to their truth status, but with a consensus that certain data and/or theories are more useful to more of the practitioners who are entitled to participate in the debate.

- The forms of reasoning conducted in research communities as they interpret the signals from their research equipment recapitulate all the known forms of human reasoning.

- Being conducted and constructed by groups of human beings, scientific, technological, and medical practices and ideas are necessarily social and human. Because those practices and ideas are about the phenomenal world, they often, but not always, also require an engagement with that world. What constitutes a satisfactory engagement with the phenomenal world is necessarily open to debate among the practitioners.

• The definition of science is made by those who are empowered to offer resources for work they consider scientific; for example, the work funded by the National Science Foundation (NSF), Social Science Research Council (SSRC), National Institutes of Health (NIH), or National Institute of Mental Health (NIMH) is science. (From Traweek 1996, 144)

Probably the most succinct and generally agreed-upon phrase that encompasses these findings comes from Andrew Pickering: "science as culture and practice" (1995, 1). This phrase builds on and fine-tunes the more polemical claim of Bruno Latour, that "the status of a [scientific] statement depends on later statements" (1987, 27). None of these scholars means to say that "anything goes" in science. But they do mean to say that the status of accepted and legitimized scientific knowledges is determined largely by social and cultural phenomena. Not every science studies scholar would agree, but as Traweek points out, "most researchers take these statements as a sort of boring baseline of shared knowledge in the field" (1996, 144).

The wide "science as practice and culture" agreement among science studies scholars creates something of a dilemma if one wishes to take *DSM-III*'s manifest content literally. Indeed, since these science studies findings are so much at variance with the "atheoretical" received view of science, it is difficult to understand how those who "do science" (like the new psychiatry) and those who "study science" have such divergent opinions about how science works. If science studies is "right," why is it that science advocates—such as supporters of the new psychiatry—in the face of so much literature that complicates and reconsiders the standard view of science, "have such turgid notions about science, engineering, and medicine, [which are] often spoken with either an ex cathedra voice or a pounding clenched-fist-in-the-face voice?" (Traweek 1996, 145).

Unless we posit that science studies as a group is all wrong about science (and, to give a sense of the acrimony within science studies, some "realist" philosophers of science go almost this far), one answer to the question of why critical science studies findings are resisted seems to involve the way the "science" trope is used in struggles for legitimacy and power. In other words, perhaps it is not the persuasive ability of the "atheoretical" argument as much as the functional uses of the argument.

In the case of the new psychiatry, by championing a rigorously scientific theory of neutrality, psychiatrists join hands with other scientists to become what feminist science studies scholar Donna Haraway calls "modest witnesses" of nature (1997, 24). For Haraway, the scientist as modest witness is

> the legitimate and authorized ventriloquist for the object world, adding nothing from his mere opinions, from his biasing embodiment. And so he is endowed with the remarkable power to establish the facts. He bears witness: he is objective; he guarantees the clarity and purity of objects. His subjectivity is his objectivity. His narratives have a magical power—they lose all trace of their history as stories, as products of partisan projects, as contestable representations, or as constructed documents in their capacity to define the facts. The narratives become clear mirrors, fully magical mirrors, without once appealing to the transcendental or the magical. (1997, 24)

Thus, when the new psychiatrist adopts the posture of modest witness, like the scientist he emulates and imitates, he may claim: "I have nothing to do with the form this knowledge has taken. Nature made me organize it this way." In reward for accepting a "passive" position with respect to nature, the psychiatric researcher fully expects to inherit the power and authority of science.

To put it another way, through aggressive theory neutrality, psychiatric science joins with science-in-general to achieve the magical position of a "culture of no culture" (Haraway 1997, 23). By adamantly denying the theory-laden and culturally contextual dimensions of psychiatric knowledge, scientific psychiatry denies being situated in a culture. When the new "atheoretical psychiatry" presents itself as a culture of no culture, the personal interests and social biases of psychiatric researchers drop out of the picture of psychiatric knowledge. All that remains is the freestanding Truth of psychiatric research. As desirable as that position may be for the new psychiatry, the science studies literature suggests that the new psychiatry's "atheoretical" approach is vastly oversimplified. And science studies effectively drives a wedge in any "commonsense" agreement with the new scientific psychiatry's theory-neutral claims. This wedge makes room not to ask who is right, but to explore an additional theoretical option for psychiatry beyond "theory neutrality." Science studies provides enough wiggle room to consider another theoretical possibility, because science studies creates doubt about the inevitability and necessity of the new psychiatry's atheoretical stance. That is enough to proceed toward an alternative choice: theoretically informed postpsychiatry.

Fortunately, the theory of postpsychiatry does not have to come from nowhere. Humanities scholars have already amassed an extensive literature on "theory" that can be drawn from (Leitch 2001). But what is "theory" in the humanities, and how can it help? The next section and the next few chapters explore "theory" in the humanities.

Humanities Theory: Poststructuralism, Postmodernism, and Postdisciplinarity

M. Kreiswirth and M. Cheetham, in their book *Theory Between the Disciplines,* sum up the humanities engagement with "theory" as follows: "however one might look at the humanities and social sciences today, it seems quite clear that the theory wars of the 1970's and 1980's are, for the most part, over and that theory has 'triumphed.'" (1990, 1). Thus, during the same period in which psychiatry consolidated itself as "atheoretical," the humanities and social sciences, and indeed the intellectual community at large, became "theoretical" beyond redemption.

But what, more precisely, do humanities scholars mean by the term *theory*? It is surprisingly hard to describe humanities "theory," because the term tends to float alone without modifiers. "Theory of what?" you might ask, but there are no easy answers. Contemporary humanities scholars rarely add antecedent adjectives (such as in "critical theory," "literary theory," or "psychoanalytic theory"), and they no longer routinely add "theory" to compound phrases (like "theory of social action," "theory of language," etc.). Combined usages still show up, but a free-floating "theory" is more common. This floating "theory" has gradually emerged because Anglo-American humanities since the 1970s have incorporated an array of theoretical writings from European sources without clear boundaries between the humanities and social sciences. As Jonathan Culler explains, "theory" writings work as a group to provide the humanities with a keen "analysis of language, or mind, or history, or culture." In addition, they offer "persuasive accounts of textual and cultural matters" (Culler 1997, 4).

There are many ways to narrate these theory writings. Vincent Leitch, the general editor of *The Norton Anthology of Theory and Criticism,* suggests five options: leading figures, key texts, significant problems, important movements, or some mixture of these (2003, 35). Pedagogically, however, assigning labels to humanities "theory" seems to help the most.

Without labels, humanities "theory" remains too vague and creates too much confusion. Replacing the labels by pulling out recurrent thematics associated with recent theory helps highlight the kinds of literature most often relevant for humanities "theory."

The recurrent themes most associated with humanities theory that usually go unlabeled are: (1) "poststructuralism," (2) "postmodernism," and (3) "postdisciplinary critique" or "cultural studies." Theory, in other words, is poststructural, it is postmodern, and it is a form of postdisciplinary critique or cultural studies. There is nothing necessary in how this worked out. It might have worked out differently, and other terms might have ended up associated with humanities theory. But as it happened, over the past thirty years, the historically contingent play of forces in the humanities brought these elements to the forefront.

Theory is poststructural because of its intense consciousness of a poststructural perspective on language. This poststructural perspective evolves out of the work of Ferdinand de Saussure, Jacques Lacan, Jacques Derrida, and Michel Foucault, and it focuses humanities theory on two main concerns: (1) a self-reflexive awareness of the role of language in shaping knowledge and practice and (2) a consistent attempt (particularly since Foucault) to chart the effects of power relations on language usage. Poststructuralist writings and themes have become so influential in the North American humanities that such work is often synonymous with an unlabeled "theory."

In poststructuralist theory, language is no longer a transparent medium available for direct and automatic translation of world to word. Language is a concern, a problem, and an object of study in its own right. Poststructuralist theory recommends that human science scholars not focus exclusively on individual examples of meaning-making but rather pay extensive attention to the linguistic context of any human meaning practice. Poststructuralist theory helps human science scholars reconstruct the elaborate background systems of linguistic convention (and the power relations that produced these systems) that give human artifacts or practices meaning in the first place.

In addition to being poststructuralist, "theory" in the humanities is "postmodern," because, like postmodernism, theory signals a break, a rupture, or a discontinuity with modernism. This postmodern aspect of theory can be confusing because the "postmodern" trope has been multiply evoked in recent years to refer to a number of breaks with modernism: aesthetic breaks, architectural breaks, cultural breaks, societal breaks, and philosophical or knowledge breaks. All of these have rele-

vance to "theory" in the humanities, but the most important is the philosophical break. Following Jean-François Lyotard's influential mono-
graph *The Postmodern Condition: A Report on Knowledge* (1984), the term
postmodern came into the orbit of poststructuralist theory and came to
designate (in at least one of its polysemic usages) a break between modernist forms of knowledge and new postmodernist forms of knowledge.
As Lyotard explains:

> I will use the term *modern* to designate any science [or knowledge]
> that legitimates itself with reference to a metadiscourse . . . [of the
> kind that makes] explicit appeal to some grand narrative, such as
> the dialectics of Spirit, the hermeneutics of meaning, the emanci-
> pation of rational or working subject, or the creation of wealth. . . .
> Simplifying to the extreme, I define postmodern as incredulity
> toward metanarratives. (1984, xxiii–xxiv)

Modernist knowledge formations, from Lyotard's perspective, ground
themselves on a foundation of Truth through Method—like the "truth
of science" obtained through faithful application of the metanarrative of
"scientific method." In its simplest form, postmodernism is skeptical of
the absolute authority of these great modernist Truth narratives.

Postmodern theory make modernism visible as one possible "way-of-
life" with a specific set of priorities, rituals, institutions, norms, and
expectations. As a way-of-life, modernism exists among an array of possible alternatives; it is not the pinnacle of civilized progress. Postmodern
theorists would not deny that modernism brings gains along some devel-
opmental lines, but modernism does not bring purified progress. Modernism also brings a multitude of losses. Sociologist Zygmunt Bauman
eloquently states this aspect of postmodern theory:

> Postmodernity is modernity coming of age: modernity looking at
> itself at a distance rather than from the inside, making a full inven-
> tory of its gains and its losses, psychoanalyzing itself, discovering the
> intentions it never before spelled out, finding them mutually cancel-
> ing and incongruous. Postmodernity is modernity coming to terms
> with its own impossibility; a self-monitoring modernity, one that con-
> sciously discards what it was unconsciously doing. (1990, 272)

In many ways, Bauman's quote perfectly captures the spirit of this book,
and his version of postmodernism (his antiutopian emphasis on trade-

offs, tough choices, and irreducible conflicts) captures the essence of theorized postpsychiatry. This form of postmodernism does not reject modernism; it only opens it up to foundational questions and alternative possibilities.

Finally, in addition to theory's poststructural and postmodern concerns, theory in the humanities is a form of postdisciplinary critique frequently given the label "cultural studies." Theory evokes a rising trend in humanities and certain social-science writing—what Richard Rorty has called a "new genre" and what Clifford Geertz has called a "blurred genre"—that borrows and intermingles ideas and methods from multiple disciplines to analyze, critique, and ultimately politicize complex disciplinary phenomena not easily reached from within a single disciplinary perspective (Rorty 1982, 66; Geertz 1973, 19). This happened because the self-consciousness that marks theory as poststructural and postmodern reflects back not only on the objects of the humanities but also on the very disciplines of the humanities. The result is that previously stable and accepted disciplinary definitions, categories, and boundaries themselves became objects of intense debate and controversy.

The most common designation of "theory" as postdisciplinary critique is the label "cultural studies." Indeed, some argue that theory ended up creating a "cultural studies" paradigm shift for the humanities. I have much more to say about cultural studies in chapter 5, but here I just want to give a sense of how the "theoretical" legacy of the last twenty years changed the very nature of humanities scholarship. Anthony Easthope argues that the crisis in representation and knowledge ushered in by "theory" created a crisis for the humanities, which transformed the field into something else: "cultural studies." Easthope argues that the older paradigm of the humanities "collapsed" through the critiques of theory and that "a fresh paradigm" of cultural studies emerged in its place. "Cultural studies'" status as a paradigm is revealed, for Easthope, "because we can more or less agree on its terms and the use of them" (1991, 5). As Easthope puts it, although pre-theory and pre–cultural studies work remains the institutional dominant in the Anglo-American context, the leading emergent edge in the humanities follows the trajectory from theory to cultural studies.

The advantage of a new theoretically informed cultural studies paradigm is that it greatly opens up previous methodological restraints. As cultural studies scholar Lawrence Grossberg puts it, "Cultural studies is an attempt to answer Marvin Gaye's question 'What is going on?' and theory is its tool to get a bit further along in the task" (1997, 4). In other words, theory helps keep disciplinary approaches open and allows scholars to ask questions based on historical and strategic needs rather than predetermined disciplinary constraints. And it allows the conceptual and methodological tools used to depend on the kinds of questions asked rather than on some preestablished methodological criteria. When scholars uncritically adopt standard disciplinary questions and methods, they place inquiry in a straitjacket (and a quiet room) before it begins. This happens because the very disciplinary methods and practices used (and the distinctions, priorities, and rituals they inscribe) too often carry within them a heritage of the investments, exclusions, and social effects that inquiry is attempting to analyze.

Another dimension of the overlap between "theory" and "cultural studies" involves the co-occurrence of political critique as key to both. As Kreiswirth and Cheetham point out, the signifiers "theory" and "critique" have become ubiquitously co-occurrent in recent academic debates and are used practically interchangeably in conferences, books, institutes, and papers (1990, 2). "Theory" as a new critical genre, as a postdisciplinary critique, is increasingly critical of historical and ideological domination and oppression as well. In "Triumph of Theory," humanities scholar J. H. Miller argues that theory has become particularly attuned to "history, culture, society, politics, institutions, class and gender conditions, the social context, the material base in the sense of institutionalization, conditions of production, technology, distribution, and consumption of 'cultural products,' among other products" (1987, 283). Theory, as Judith Butler puts it, works to enhance its political salience in "the context of politically invested arenas—race, colonialism, sexuality, gender—[that] are generally situated within a left of academic discourse" (Butler, Guillory, and Thomas 2000, ix).

Likewise, "cultural studies" scholars understand their work as both an intellectual practice and a political tradition. As L. Grossberg, C. Nelson, and P. Treichler put it, "cultural studies" is not only the ground on which analysis proceeds but also the site of a political critique:

> In virtually all traditions of cultural studies, its practitioners see cultural studies not simply as a chronicle of cultural change but as an intervention in it, and see themselves not simply as scholars providing an account but as politically engaged participants. (1992, 5)

Cultural studies of science practitioner Donna Haraway echoes this sentiment when she says, "The point is to make a difference in the world, to cast our lot for some ways of life and not others" (1997, 36). Or, in another of Haraway's poetic incantations: "The point is to learn to remember that we might have been otherwise, and might yet be, as a matter of embodied fact" (1997, 39).

In conclusion to this section, my review of humanities theory has not provided a foundational definition of "theory," nor has it discovered the "Truth of Theory." Instead, it weaves a garland of meanings out of the many thematic connotations that have been associated with recent theory in the humanities. Theory in the humanities is poststructural, it is postmodern, and it is a kind postdisciplinary cultural studies critique. The main effect of this kind of theory, as Culler argues, "is the disputing of 'common sense' . . . views about . . . meaning, writing, literature, experience" (1997, 4). For Culler, theory questions

> the conception that the meaning of an utterance or text is what the speaker "had in mind," or the idea that writing is an expression whose truth lies elsewhere, in an experience or a state of affairs which it expresses, or the notion that reality is what is "present" at any given moment. (1997, 4)

Theory provides the humanities with powerful tools and opportunities for breaking away from commonsense modernist disciplinary practices, and theory provides the humanities with a nuanced understanding of the role of language and power in the shaping of knowledge.

Postpsychiatric Studies, or "Theorizing Psychiatry"

Out of this swirl of "theoretical" activity in the humanities, my proposal for reinvigorating psychiatric studies emerges and takes shape. An alternative theorized postpsychiatry that engages itself with the humanities— indeed, a branch of psychiatry that maintains its connections with general intellectual thought—would be a postpsychiatric alternative that accepts and seriously wrestles with theory. A theorized postpsychiatry would allow itself to be decentered and dislocated from its increasingly settled path. It would address rather than efface the multiple determinations, besides objective Truth, of the currently leading representations of psychiatric knowledge. A theorized postpsychiatry would, in the words of Edward Said, wrestle with "the fact that a representation is *eo ipso* implicated, intertwined, embedded, interwoven with a great many other things besides the 'truth,' which is itself a representation" (1978, 272). Once this idea is fully understood, it will seem impossible, at least for some in the psychiatric community, to go back to the rhetoric of "atheo-retical" psychiatry.

Rather than conform to the new scientific psychiatry or nostalgically return to psychoanalysis, a theorized postpsychiatry would draw on resources from poststructuralism, postmodernism, and cultural studies. Postpsychiatry would be *poststructural* in that it would take seriously the role of language and power in shaping psychiatric thought and perception, and it would devote as many resources to working through theories of language and power as the new psychiatry currently spends on working through statistical science and neuropharmacology. Postpsychiatry would be *postmodern* in that it would work without the pseudo-foundations and pseudo-certainties of modernist science and reason. For postpsychiatry, key values of the clinical encounter would include not only the modernist values of empirical diagnosis and rational therapeutics but also additional clinical values like ethics, aesthetics, humor, empathy, kindness, and justice.

Finally, postpsychiatry would be a form of *cultural studies* as it would embrace postdisciplinary and multidisciplinary scholarship and methodologies. Rather than drawing exclusively from the medical sciences and neurosciences, postpsychiatry would join with the humanities, the arts, the social sciences, and an array of critical postdisciplinary programs like disability studies, gender studies, postcolonial studies, gay and lesbian studies, and so on. These postdisciplinary alignments would allow psychiatry to join and form coalitions with the rest of the academy. Rigid disciplinary boundaries cause tremendous limitations in any form of scholarship, but psychiatry (the quintessential human concern) cut off from the humanities and critical postdisciplinary programs is absurd. Postpsychiatry would reverse the absurdity of this scholarly imbalance.

It is important to note that these changes must be more than changes taken by individual psychiatrists. These changes must affect the field as a whole. The challenge is not for individual psychiatrists to be more "broad-minded." The challenge is for psychiatric journals, texts, courses, conferences, research, and education as a whole to be much more interconnected with intellectual thought beyond today's current clinical sciences. That being said, of course, it is also possible for individual psychiatrists to make moves in these directions. And when they succeed, all the better. But for this kind of change to meaningfully affect the standards of care within clinics will require psychiatry as a whole either to change or to tolerate a significant branch or subsection of itself being more intellectually diverse. That will necessitate a substantial shift from the psychiatric discipline we know today.

CHAPTER TWO

Dodging the Science Wars

A Theoretical Third Way

Unfortunately, psychiatric studies cannot theorize itself, and postpsychiatry cannot emerge without running into the science wars. Science warriors vehemently attack every kind of scholarship I recommended in the last chapter—poststructuralism, postmodernism, cultural studies, science studies, and even humanities theory itself. These science warriors warn that theory is a threat to public trust and to public funding for science. Most of all, they warn that theory will unleash a new era of superstition and quackery. Science fundamentalists Paul Gross and Norman Levitt initiated the science wars with a preemptive strike they entitled *Higher Superstition: The Academic Left and Its Quarrels with Science* (1994), and their work continues to shape the struggles and the fighting.[1] Gross and Levitt do not see recent humanities theory as an important corrective to the hubris of reason and science. Rather, they see recent work in the humanities as consisting of dangerous theories of mass destruction, and they have set out to rid the university of these hazardous conceptual weapons.

Gross and Levitt use polemic strategies to devastate and demoralize their opponents. They call humanities theory "muddleheaded," "sheer puffery," "a swarm of silly errors," and a "fog of philosophical conceits" (1994, 246). They charge that theory scholarship ranges in quality from "seriously flawed to hopelessly flawed" and is an "intellectual debility afflicting the contemporary university" (1994, 41, 7). Beyond these polemics, Gross and Levitt's only real argument against theory scholarship centers on what they consider its "relativist" or "cultural constructivist" approaches to science (1994, 50). The "central tenet" of relativist critiques, according to Gross and Levitt, is that scientific discoveries are not objective representations of the world. Relativists, according to Gross and Levitt, see science as "the expression of 'local truths' or 'structures' that make sense only within a certain context of social experience and a certain political symbology" (1994, 38). Relativists miss what Gross and Levitt think should be obvious: the "universality, timelessness, and uncontextual validity of science" (1994, 38). Gross and Levitt make this argument by drawing a sharp distinction between realism and relativism. They take sides with the realists, and they wage war against muddle-headed relativists of all stripes. Their work has set up the either/or battle lines that continue to shape the science wars.

Influential new psychiatrists have picked up and mimicked Gross and Levitt's science-war rhetoric. Sally Satel, for example, the current psychiatric advisor to the George Walker Bush administration, cites Gross and Levitt favorably in her diatribe against humanities theory entitled *PC, M.D.: How Political Correctness Is Corrupting Medicine*. She calls theory an "ideological staple of the humanities, fine arts, and social studies," and she alleges that if theory takes hold in medicine and psychiatry it will badly corrupt standards of excellence and professionalism (2000, 11, 233). Like Gross and Levitt, Satel raises the specter of superstition and quackery: theory risks "dumbing down the curriculum, teaching pseudo-science, and promoting feel-good, unproven remedies" (2000, 100). Satel does not make arguments for these claims; she simply rides on the relativist arguments already worked out in *Higher Superstition*.

Like many who have responded to the science wars, I object to the controversy's basic premises.[2] Although there is some merit in Gross and Levitt's discussion of the difference between realism and relativism, their attacks make it hard to sustain a meaningful dialogue. They overdramatize the problems with relativism, and they overstate the value of realism. Most of all, they imply that there is no way out of the realism/relativism binary—except to take sides and fight.

Postpsychiatry must develop third-way approaches to sidestep such science-wars hostilities. Third-way approaches could be drawn from an array of different scholarships—the philosophy of science, science studies, feminist and cultural studies of science. I believe one of the best approaches is to draw from contemporary humanities theory to develop a deep appreciation of the complexities of psychiatric representation. The poststructuralist strand in humanities theory repeatedly emphasizes the inevitable linguistic mediation of all knowledge representation (including in science). By developing a broader understanding of how representation works, postpsychiatry can avoid the either/or polemics of the science wars.

Theories of representation begin with the recognition that representational languages are inevitably composed of signs. Representational languages, including scientific ones, use signs to stand for (or represent) thoughts, concepts, ideas, or feelings. Spoken languages use sounds, written languages use words, visual languages use images, fashion languages use clothing, body languages use gestures, and facial languages use arrangements of facial features. All these signifying elements, or signs, form the fundamental building blocks of communication and performative interaction. In each case, the elements of a language—sounds, words, images, clothing, gestures, or facial features—construct meaning and transmit it. They signify. They carry meaning because they operate as signs.

Signs, however, are complex, and there have been several "philosophies of the sign." In this chapter, I look in detail at three philosophic approaches to the sign: (1) referential, (2) relational, and (3) pragmatic. The referential approach has largely been developed by Anglo-American philosophy, the relational approach by Continental philosophy, and the pragmatic approach by American pragmatism. Each philosophic approach to the sign creates an alternative ontology and an alternative epistemology. By *ontology*, I refer to the broad underlying assumptions people have about the world's core existential features. Alternative ontologies create very different notions of the world's content and the world's core features. By *epistemology*, I refer to the broad underlying assumptions people have about knowledge acquisition and proper knowledge legitimization. Alternative epistemologies create very different assumptions about proper methodological approaches to knowledge. Together, alternative ontologies and epistemologies structure very different perspectives (or logics of common sense) with regard to the world and knowledge. When commonsense logics differ enough, they create the grounds for protracted conflict—like that demonstrated in the science wars.

Schematically, the three approaches to the sign I consider (along with their implied ontologies and epistemologies) look like this:

Theory of the sign	*Ontology*	*Epistemology*
1. referential	realism	correspondence
2. relational	relativism	social construction
3. pragmatic	semiotic realism	pluridemensional consequences

Reference theories of the sign, then, tend toward realist ontology and a correspondence epistemology. Relational theories of the sign tend toward relativist ontology and a social-construction epistemology. And pragmatic theories of the sign tend toward an ontology of semiotic realism and an epistemology of pluridemensional consequences. When these three approaches to the sign are taken together (rather than set in conflict with each other) and then applied to psychiatry, they create a nimble and nuanced theory of psychiatric representation—nimble and nuanced enough to help postpsychiatry avoid being shot down in the science wars.

Referential Theories of the Sign

Science warriors like Gross and Levitt base their confident realism on a referential theory of the sign. Referential theories of the sign come in two primary forms: commonsense versions and detailed philosophic versions. Westerners, including most Western-influenced psychiatrists, tend toward commonsense versions. Anglo-American philosophers tend toward philosophic versions. The philosophic versions build on the nineteenth-century work of the philosopher Gottlob Frege (1952). For both the commonsense and the philosophic versions, signs work through reference and reference determines meaning.

In a reference theory of the sign, signs get their meaning by standing for, or indicating, something in the world. The sign and the object are in a dyadic relationship with one another. The sign *tree* signifies because it stands for a concrete object: a tree. This same pattern holds for abstract ideas. For a reference theory, abstract signs like *freedom* or *psychosis* signify because they too refer to something in the world that exists independent of human representational tags. For example, the fact that some people are "free" and some are "psychotic," while others are not, depends on actual features of the world. For a reference theory, whether a "tree" is real, or whether people really are "free" or "psychotic," does not depend on what people say about these things. Nor does it depend on people's conceptual categories or their interpretive traditions. The primary determinate of a sign is based on on objective facts of the world independent of these human concerns.

Referential theory is the dominant theory in psychiatry. To see it at work, consider the following claim by new psychiatrists Richard Wyatt and Kay Jamison. These biopsychiatry advocates use a referential approach to retrospectively diagnose Vincent Van Gogh with "manic-depressive illness." Van Gogh, they claim, had manic-depressive illness because he exhibited the following real-world features:

psychiatric symptoms (extreme mood changes, including long periods of depression and extended episodes of highly active, volatile and excited states, altered sleep patterns, hyperreligiosity, extreme irritability, visual and auditory hallucinations, violence, agitation, and alcohol abuse), the age of onset of his symptoms (late adolescence, early twenties), his premorbid personality, the cyclic nature of his attacks, which were interspersed with long periods of highly lucid functioning, the lack of intellectual deterioration over time, the increasing severity of his mood swings, the seasonal exacerbation in his symptoms, and his quite remarkable family history of suicide and psychiatric illness. (Jamison 1993, 141)

Using a commonsense reference theory, Wyatt and Jamison see these "real-world" facts as determining the truth about Van Gogh.

If we put Wyatt and Jamison's claim in the language of Anglo-American philosophy, the truth conditions for a sentence like "Vincent Van Gogh had manic-depressive illness" may be expressed in terms of reference as follows:

> "Vincent Van Gogh had manic-depressive illness" is true if and only if (a) there is some object that "Vincent Van Gogh" designates and (b) "manic-depressive illness" applies to that object.

There are two distinct reference relations in this sentence: (a) *designation*—holding between the name "Vincent Van Gogh" and an object; and (b) *application*—holding between the predicate "manic-depressive illness" and many objects, manic-depressive ones (Devitt and Sterelny 1993, 18). For the sentence to be true, it must refer to a Vincent Van Gogh who was actually manic-depressive. Nothing else is needed. It is irrelevant whether Van Gogh was ever diagnosed as manic-depressive, ever considered himself to be manic-depressive, or would have wanted his life interpreted in that way.

Though reference theories of the sign dominate in Western minds, reference theory has been the source of much philosophic debate and controversy (for a discussion, see Devitt and Sterelny 1993). Instead of going into the details of these philosophic controversies, however, I want to focus on the larger ontological and epistemological implications that generally follow from referential theories of the sign. Science warriors like Gross and Levitt do not speak in terms of theories of the sign. They attack humanities theory on the grounds of their confident realist ontology and their correspondence epistemology. But the confidence they place in their ontology and epistemology does not come from actual reference to the world, from something like the "force of nature." Rather, it comes from their assumed reference theory of the sign.

To see Gross and Levitt's ontological realism at work and its connection with their assumed reference theory of the sign, we have to articulate their form of realism. Gross and Levitt do not explicitly define their realism, but it is not hard to see their perspective in philosopher Hillary Putnam's definition: "A realist (with respect to a given theory or discourse) holds that 1.) sentences of that theory are true or false; and 2.) that what makes them true or false is something external—that is to say, not our sense data, . . . the structure of our minds, or our language" (1975, 69). This definition of realism relies on a reference theory of the sign. Meaning is created by something outside the sign in the external world, independent of what anyone might say or think about it.

Gross and Levitt's assumed reference theory of the sign also backs up their confident correspondence epistemology. In a correspondence theory of knowledge, the truth of a sign depends on its correspondence with the actual world. In a correspondence theory, concerns like tradition, authority, intuition, emotions, and desire are largely irrelevant in determining truth. A correspondence theory would say, "Don't tell me about your artistic intuitions regarding Van Gogh's paintings, don't tell me what his contemporaries said, and don't tell me what artistic historians and traditions say about him. Just tell me the facts! Did Van Gogh meet the criteria for the disorder or not?" The only thing that matters in a correspondence theory of truth is whether there is a direct correspondence with the actual world.

Relational Theories of the Sign

Science warriors like Gross and Levitt favor realism because they dramatically fear that constructivist alternatives yield the chaos of relativism. They treat constructivism and relativism as wildly muddleheaded and derelict. But constructivism is not so muddleheaded as all that, and postpsychiatry should not approach constructivism with such blunt polemics. Postpsychiatry scholars can best give constructivist alternatives a legitimate hearing, and thereby go beyond the science wars, by seriously considering the theory of representation on which the most powerful constructivist versions rest. The most powerful version comes from structural linguist Ferdinand de Saussure. In the late nineteenth century, Saussure developed a relational theory of the sign that has gone on to be the major stimulus for poststructuralist philosophy.

To understand Saussure, we have to define some terms. Saussure focused his theory of the sign on the dyadic relationship between the *signifier* and the *signified.* The *signifier* is something that signifies, like a word. The *signified* is that which the signifier represents. For Saussure, the signified is not an object but a concept. Saussure's definitional focus represents a major break with reference theory. Reference theory concentrates on the dyadic connection between the signifier and the object, but Saussure concentrates on the dyadic connection between the signifier and the concept. This focus completely reverses the direction of reference theory. Where reference theory concentrates on objects found in the world, Saussure's theory concentrates on concepts found inside people's heads and in their linguistic, or semiotic, communities. The results of these alternative focuses could not be more different.

For Saussure, the signifier *tree* stands for, or indicates, the *concept* of a tree (not the *object* of a tree). In sharp contrast to reference theory, Saussure argues that the concept of a tree is distinguished from the concept of a bush (or a vine, or a pole, or an oak, or a giraffe) not through referential features of the object itself but through relational semiotic features of the concept in comparison with other concepts. As Saussure puts it, "the mechanism of language turns entirely on identities and differences . . . [with no] element of imposition from the outside world" (1972, 118). In other words, for Saussure, a language works through internal semiotic relations and not through external reference—which is why I call Saussure's theory a *relational theory of the sign.*

A relational theory of the sign is possible, Saussure argues, because language prestructures meaning through a system of semiotic differences without positive terms:

> A linguistic system is a series of phonetic differences matched with a series of conceptual differences. This matching of a certain number of auditory signals and a similar number of items carved out from the mass of thought gives rise to a system of values. It is this system which provides the operative bond between phonic and mental elements within each sign. (1972, 118)

Language can work without reference for Saussure because speakers use a relational semiotic grid of signifiers (rather than references) to communicate with each other. The relational grid differentiates signifiers and concepts from one another and allows communication with other speakers who have access to a similar semiotic grid of signifiers and concepts. As a result, linguistic communication can occur independent of reference. Communicators do not need actual unicorns to know what the signifier *unicorn* means or to differentiate between a *unicorn* and a *leprechaun*. This insight into linguistic functioning changes everything.

French poststructuralist philosophers built on Saussure's relational theory to introduce what science warriors call a radical social-constructionist approach to reason and science.[3] The details and intricacies of poststructuralist thought are complex and controversial. But for our purposes, the most important thing to note is that poststructuralism brings out the radical ontological and epistemological implications of Saussure's relational theory of the sign. As poststructural philosopher Michel Foucault playfully describes it, Saussure's relational theory of the sign opens the door to a deep appreciation of the "truth" in a fictional tale by Jorge Luis Borges. The Borges tale speaks of an imaginary Chinese encyclopedia with strange and unusual passages. Foucault puts it this way:

> This passage quotes a certain Chinese encyclopedia in which it is written that animals are divided into: "(a) belonging to the Emperor, (b) embalmed, (c) tame, (d) suckling pigs, (e) sirens, (f) fabulous, (g) stray dogs, (h) included in present classification, (i) frenzied, (j) innumerable, (k) drawn with a very fine camelhair brush, (l) et cetera, (m) having just broken the water pitcher, (n) that from a long way off look like flies." In the wonderment of this taxonomy, the thing we apprehend in one great leap, the thing that, by means of this fable, is demonstrated as the exotic charm of another system of thought, is the limitation of our own, the stark impossibility of thinking that. (1970, xv)

Foucault's revelation here, his radical insight, is none other than the stark impossibility of a purely referential theory of language. If all systems of thought and their linguistic classificatory schemas work through semiotic relations rather than reference—analogous to Borges's Chinese encyclopedia—there is an inescapable silliness at the core of all referential pretensions.

Putting relational theories of the sign in terms of ontology and epistemology, we can see that relational theories of the sign tend toward relativist ontology and social-constructionist epistemology. A relativist ontology is most consistent with relational theories of the sign because, in relational theories, signs work not by referring to the real world but by connecting and differentiating conceptual categories in order to allow communication. Similarly, relational theories of the sign tend toward a social-constructionist epistemology because constraint on belief comes from consistency with and differentiation from other beliefs rather than from correspondence with the world. Truth is checked not by its correspondence to the world but by its relational connections with conceptual categories. As such, social-constructionist epistemology draws much of its strength from tradition, authority, and politics.

In the psychiatry example from the last section, a relativist ontology and constructionist epistemology seriously complicate Wyatt and Jamison's referential diagnosis of Vincent Van Gogh. From a relational perspective, the claim that Van Gogh had manic-depressive illness depends less on the referent and more on the socially constructed categories and conceptual grids used by different interpretive communities. From this view, there would be no "single" truth of Van Gogh. When interpreters coming from diverse semiotic communities apply their respective categories and systems of thought (according to the rules and norms of their respective communities), they create multiple "true" interpretations. Unlike the science warriors, relational theorists do not see this as an aberration to be attacked; they see it as an inevitability to be appreciated. Relational theorists do not see chaos; they see the possibility of alternative interpretations and the need to respect alternative worldviews.

The relational perspective of multiple and alternative interpretations has a critical value that gets lost in the science-wars polemics. Van Gogh's life, like all lives, was extremely complicated. Reducing the "truth" of Van Gogh's life to a single interpretation loses this complexity. Indeed, the many interpretations people have made of Van Gogh's life create a particularly rich example of multiple possibilities. In my reading, interpreters of Van Gogh fall into two broad traditions: those who pathologize him and those who celebrate him.[4]

The pathologizers are primarily clinical writers, and they may be further broken down into two main categories: those grounded in biopsychiatry and those grounded in psychology. Biopsychiatry interpretations of Van Gogh (e.g., Wyatt and Jamison) are differentiated along an interpretive grid that includes bipolar disorder, unipolar depression, schizophrenia, schizoaffective disorder, temporal lobe epilepsy, tertiary syphilis, and porphorea (just to name a few). Psychological interpretations are differentiated along a grid that includes depression, obsession, masochism, personality disorder, replacement child syndrome, and existential despair. The two clinical communities dramatically disagree on how to match their respective categorical grids with Van Gogh's life. But they both agree that Van Gogh was "sick" and that his mental pathology explains his psychic suffering and much of his artistic innovation.

In sharp contrast, celebratory interpreters argue that Van Gogh did not live a pathological life—he lived an inspirational one. Celebratory interpreters consider Van Gogh's life one of extraordinary courage, conviction, and sacrifice. For them, Van Gogh's struggles indicate his intense willingness to sacrifice for humanity and for art. These interpreters also disagree on the specifics—particularly on the different motives for Van Gogh's sacrifice. But they agree on the basic interpretive frame. The relational grid they work from falls out along motivational categories of aesthetics, spirituality, social inequality, or a nexus of all three. In other words, celebratory interpreters disagree on whether Van Gogh's sacrificial quest was primarily aesthetic, spiritual, or political, but they all agree that his genius allowed him to make major progress on fundamental human concerns despite tremendous cost to himself. For these interpreters, we should not pathologize Van Gogh; we should learn from him. We should not "cure" him; we should let him cure us.

As Henri Nouwen puts it in his reflections on Van Gogh, "I have never found students more personally, intellectually, and emotionally involved than they were during periods of attentive looking at Vincent's drawings and paintings. I still remember how we would spend long hours together in silence, simply gazing at the slides of Vincent's work" (1989, x). Van Gogh, the ever sorrowful yet always rejoicing Dutch painter, helped Nouwen and his students tune in to "the deepest yearnings of their souls." Nouwen describes it this way:

The hours spent walking through the Kroller-Moller Museum in the Netherlands and the days spent reading [Van Gogh's] letters were personal times of restoration and renewal. They were times of solitude in which a voice spoke I could listen to. I experienced connections between Vincent's struggle and my own, and realized more and more that Vincent was becoming my wounded healer. He painted what I had not before dared to look at; he questioned what I had not before dared to speak about; and he entered into spaces of the heart that I had not before dared to come close to. (1989, x)

Nouwen celebrates Van Gogh rather than pathologizing him. Indeed, Van Gogh's courageous struggles so inspired Nouwen that he became the "main spiritual guide" of Nouwen's life (1989, x).

From a relational perspective, these multiple interpretations of Van Gogh are not a problem, and they are not muddleheaded or derelict. Alternative interpretations of Van Gogh's life are simply the result of the relativism that comes from alternative social constructions. When people apply different relational grids to Van Gogh's life, they come up with different interpretations. From a relational perspective, this insight does not lead to chaos so much as it helps people understand the need to tolerate interpretive diversity.

Pragmatic Theories of the Sign

The third theory of the sign I consider here comes from the American pragmatic tradition. In the late nineteenth century, contemporaneous with Frege and Saussure, the American philosopher and founder of pragmatism, Charles Sanders Peirce, also developed a theory of the sign. Unlike the dyadic theories of Frege and Saussure, Peirce's theory is triadic. Peirce saw the sign as a three-way relationship between the concept (interpretant), the signifier (sign), and the thing (object). For Peirce, signs must be interpreted by tacking back and forth between all three parts of the sign. He sharply critiqued both referential and relational theories of the sign. With regard to reference theories, Peirce argued that perhaps in plants there might be a dyadic theory of the sign that focused on the referent. A sunflower turning toward the sun might rely on reference independent of conceptual relations, but Peirce argued that such a theory was highly implausible for human representation. With regard to relational theory, Peirce argued that a human dyadic theory of the sign that focused only on conceptual relations but conveyed no information about the world was "very strange" (1955, 100). He wondered how people using a relational theory could ever negotiate the world.

Peirce stressed that all dyadic approaches to the sign are incomplete: "the triadic relation is genuine, that is its three members are bound together by it in a way that does not consist in any complexus of dyadic relations" (1955, 100). "All [human] thought . . . must necessarily be in signs," and all signs are simultaneously connected to both interpretants *and* objects (1991b, 49). The advantage of Peirce's triadic theory of the sign is that it provides greater flexibility than either a referential or a relational theory of the sign because it incorporates insights from both theories. For Peirce, signs have meaning both because they are referential and because they are relational. They connect both to the world and to the linguistic system from which they arise.

The simultaneously referential and relational aspects of Peirce's theory can be better understood by analyzing his distinctions among signs. Peirce classified signs into three categories:

1. The *icon* is a sign that refers to the object through its likeness or similarity to it. For example, a sketch of a tree represents the tree by resembling it.
2. The *index* conveys the object by being effected by it; thus a weathercock is an index of the wind.
3. The *symbol* refers to an object that it designates by a sort of law, by convention, or by habit of connection. Most words, for example, are symbols.

The referential aspects of Peirce's theory are most obvious in his categories of icon and index. In these categories, reference to the real world, either through resemblance or through effect, connects the sign directly with the object. By contrast, the relational aspects of Peirce's theory are more prominent in his category of symbols. Symbols are arbitrary, determined by semiotic convention. As in Saussure's theory of the sign, though much less worked out in Peirce, symbols work by differentiating concepts from one another.

However, and this is key for Peirce, none of the categories works entirely by reference or relation alone. Icons and indexes are interpreted not only by their reference to objects but also by normative rules of interpretation in a given community. The standard icon for a tree—a line with a triangle on top—does not really look like a tree, and a weathercock does not really say anything transparent about the wind without a whole series of conventions on how to interpret it. Thus, though icons and indexes work through reference, conventionality is also necessary for meaning.

The opposite is true for symbols. Symbols are interpreted not by conventional semiotic relations alone but also through reference. Peirce calls reference the "ground" of a sign. Even with symbols, signs do not purely relate to conceptual ideas. Even a symbol "stands for something, its object. It stands for that object, not in all respects, but in reference to a sort of idea, which I have sometimes called the ground of the representamen" (Peirce 1955, 99). For Peirce, symbolic representations of the real world are not merely representations but also predictions of future events. As such, symbols can never be determined by our ideas alone but are also determined by reference to our experiences with the real world:

> When I say that really to be is different from being represented, I mean that what really is ultimately consists in what shall be forced upon us in experience, that there is an element of brute compulsion in fact and that fact is not a mere question of reasonableness. (Peirce 1991a, 243)

Thus, even with symbols, where Peirce most clearly relies on a relational semiotic interpretation, meaning is partly determined by reference to experience of the world.

Pragmatic theories of the sign are most consistent with an ontology I call "semiotic realism" and an epistemology of "pluridimensional consequences." An ontology of semiotic realism suggests that there is a real world out there that "grounds our ideas" or that our ideas are "in touch with." At the same time, the specific points of contact between our ideas and the world are determined by the semiotic relations from which our ideas are structured. These semiotic relations are relative to a given community or a specific tradition of thought. Semiotic realism rejects an ontology of either realism or constructivism because it contains insights from both. From a semiotic-realist perspective, ideas are grounded in the real world, but how and why they are grounded remains relative to diverse semiotic communities.

The pragmatic epistemology of "pluridimensional consequences" takes off from there. I borrow the term *pluridimensional* not from the pragmatists but from French linguist Roland Barthes. The phrase "pluridimensional order" articulates for Barthes the way that specific languages always remain too limited to capture the world in total (Barthes 1982, 465). Despite this limitation of language, all linguistic communities do evoke, engage, and negotiate the world through some element of grounding or contact. Language, therefore, contains both referential and relational elements. Languages do not fully mirror or correspond to the world in all of the world's complexity, but languages do make real connections with the world.

Different connections with the world yield different *consequences* for practice and lived experience. These consequences are key for pragmatic theories. Indeed, the epistemology of pragmatic theories of the sign focuses the judgment of what is good knowledge specifically on the criterion of consequences. Where reference theories focus knowledge evaluators on correspondence, and relational theories focus knowledge evaluators on socially constructed traditions, pragmatic theories focus knowledge evaluators on consequences for action. The focus on consequences arises from the pragmatic perspective that knowledge functions as a guide for practical action. Thus, the best knowledge is that which leads to the best consequences in practice. This consequentialist perspective is the most comprehensive of the three philosophies of the sign because the pragmatic focus does not erase the importance of either correspondence or social construction as criteria for knowledge. Rather, pragmatic consequential epistemology incorporates both correspondence and construction because good consequences depend partly on correspondence with experience and partly on relations with community and tradition.

Unique to consequential epistemology's focus on consequences is its orientation toward the future. Consequential epistemology measures good representations based on what will happen next, not on what has happened before. This future orientation means that consequential epistemology is unique in its incorporation of values and desire into epistemology. In construction or correspondence epistemologies, human desire has nothing to do with truth. The "true" from these epistemologies depends either on correspondence independent of people or on coherence with constructed communities. In a consequential epistemology, desired consequences are part of what determines best belief. If two beliefs seem equally plausible based on grounds of reference and grounds of tradition, but one has better consequences than the other, then the one with best consequences is the one to choose. By including desire in belief evaluation, consequential epistemology reconnects beliefs with values. Rather than separating ontology and epistemology from ethical values, it brings them together. Consequential epistemology reconnects ontological questions (e.g., "What are the core aspects of people?") and epistemological questions (e.g., "What is the best way to gain knowledge about people?") with ethical questions (e.g., "What kind of people do we want to be?" and "What kind of life-worlds do we want to create?").

In psychiatry, different understandings of the core features of people and different approaches to inquiry about people yield very different kinds of people described and discovered. They also yield very different kinds of life experiences. That's where the phrase "pluridimensional consequences" comes together. The epistemology of pragmatism simultaneously considers that there are many possible ways to organize human life and that differentiation among these different ways depends partly on consequences and desired values. In other words, there are multiple paths to wisdom. There are many ways to ground the world that will lead to "good hours." Indeed, the grandfather of pragmatism, Ralph Waldo Emerson, defines "wisdom" as a plenitude of "good hours." For Emerson, "to finish the moment, to find the journey's end in every step of the road, to live the greatest number of good hours, [that] is wisdom. . . . The only ballast I know is a respect to the present hour" (1946, 274). The ballast of the present hour is a ballast that can only be reached with an epistemology of pluridimensional consequences. If there is a pluridimensional variety of ways to organize the world, then many of these ways could lead to good hours. Which way to choose depends not only on correspondence to the world or on constructed traditions. It also depends on desired consequences.

Before going further, I should point out that although I use Peirce's pragmatic theory of the sign to help organize my ontology of semiotic realism and my epistemology of pluridimensional consequences, Peirce's writings themselves do not reliably support these notions. Accordingly, the version of Peirce I am using must be considered a modified version. In the first of Peirce's classic articles on pragmatism, "The Fixation of Belief," Peirce sounds very much the robust (rather than semiotic) realist, and he argues forcefully that no matter what we may believe about the world there can be "only one true conclusion" that is real (1982a, 74). However, in a later article, "How to Make Our Ideas Clear," Peirce is more equivocal about this, grounding "truth" and "reality" in a more social-constructionist phrase: "The opinion which is fated to be ultimately agreed to by all who investigate" (1982b, 97). But even by this phrase, Peirce seems to mean that if investigation were carried out long enough, the final opinion would be a single truth, not multiple ones.

There is nothing necessary in following Peirce's insistence on single truths. Indeed, if the symbolic (or relational) part of Peirce's theory of the sign is modeled along the lines of Saussure's semiotic work, I think pluridimensional truths are more consistent. When investigators work within differing language practices, they come up with different linguistic formations to preoccupy them and to organize their life (and their world). Therefore, I will sidestep Peirce's version of robust realism by simply taking fellow pragmatist William James's tack: I will reinterpret Peirce against the grain of his own intentions. James interprets Peirce as providing a theory of the sign that creates a space for both realism and a plurality of social constructions of the real—in other words, semiotic realism and pluridimensional consequences.

For James, there cannot be one truth because all truth is instrumental. Beliefs are more analogous to tools than to copies of reality. Like tools, beliefs help us cope with the world, and coping is more important for James than are abstract notions like correspondence. James may be understood as a pluridimensionalist in that he does not deny that there is a world independent of humans or that the world impinges on human sensations. But for James, how we understand the independent world, or how we interpret its impingement on our sensations, depends on our perspectives and our interpretive communities:

> Which [sensation] we attend to, note, and make emphatic in our conclusions depends on our own interests; and according as we lay the emphasis here or there, quite different formulations of truth result. We read the same facts differently. "Waterloo," with the same fixed details, spells a "victory" for the Englishman; for a Frenchman it spells a "defeat." . . . What we say about reality thus depends on the perspective into which we throw it. (1992, 118)

In this example, James uses a pragmatic approach that weaves together realism (correspondence with what happened) and relativism (interpretation of what happened in terms of differentially constructed communities) to come up with what I'm calling semiotic realism. In addition, James also shows a pluridimensional-consequentialist epistemology at work. The "truth" of the Waterloo example depends partly on the interests of the knowledge makers. Interpreters' interests are based on their attendance to different aspects of the data, which means that interests, desires, and consequences partly determine what counts as legitimate knowledge.

As a result, a pragmatic theory of the sign incorporates and goes beyond both relational and reference theories of the sign. If we return to the Van Gogh example, a pragmatic approach allows interpreters the flexibility and openness of a variety of interpretations. Van Gogh's life viewed from an ontology of semiotic realism is too richly complex for any one interpretation to fully capture. At the same time, semiotic realism includes the real in that all of the Van Gogh interpretative communities have a ground in the real. But from a pragmatic perspective, no one community has exclusive rights to the real; they are all grounded in different approaches with very different consequences. From an epistemology of pluridimensional consequences, which interpretation to choose and which interpretive community to join ultimately depend on consequences and desires. Answers to questions like "What is the best way to understand Van Gogh?" and "What is the best way to generate knowledge about Van Gogh?" depend partly on answers to questions like "What kind of person would Van Gogh want to be?" and "What kind of life-world would he want to create?"

Since Van Gogh is no longer alive, these questions reflect back on the interpreters themselves. If we see our own Van Gogh–like struggles through a pathologizing light, we become a certain kind of people. If we see our Van Gogh–like struggles through a celebratory light, we become a very different kind of people. From a semiotic-realism perspective, there does not have to be a single right way to interpret Van Gogh. That does not mean, however, that there can be no differentiation among interpretations. From a pluridimensional-consequences perspective, the interpretations we choose and the knowledge-making communities we join determine who we become and the kind of life-worlds we create. Differentiating among interpretations therefore involves differentiating among the kinds of life-worlds we want and the kinds of communities we desire.

Postpsychiatry and Pragmatic Theories of the Sign

Pragmatic theories of the sign have the most to offer postpsychiatry. Pragmatic approaches bring an ontology of semiotic realism and an epistemology of pluridimensional consequences. This pragmatic ontology and epistemology allow postpsychiatry to negotiate the realism/relativism binary and the fundamental difficulties of both realism and relativism. Furthermore, pragmatic approaches are at the heart of much science studies scholarship, and they help postpsychiatry sidestep the polemics of the science wars.

As the very phenomena of the science wars make clear, both reference and relational approaches have fundamental problems. Reference approaches create a "one-truth" certainty but risk authoritarian dogmatism and intolerance. Relational approaches avoid dogmatism but risk a lack of criteria for making choices among interpretive communities. These mirroring problems become clear in the Van Gogh example.

Wyatt and Jamison—with their claim that the artist was "manic-depressive"—demonstrate a referential approach to Van Gogh's life. For them, "manic-depressive illness" becomes the necessary One Truth because Van Gogh fits the referential criteria. They believe that the term *manic-depression* corresponds to the world regardless of what anyone may think about it. Manic-depression represents "the real" of Van Gogh's life. Wyatt and Jamison make their referential claim with no mention of alternative conceptual frames or alternative traditions of interpretation. They make no mention of the consequences of this kind of psychiatric interpretation for Van Gogh, for artists in general, or for broader humanity. Since Wyatt and Jamison work with an assumed referential theory, they don't have to. The only thing that matters in making the referential claim are the "facts" of the world, independent of human concerns like interpretive traditions and human consequences.

This kind of referential certainty, even dogmatism, can all too readily slide into authoritarianism and intolerance. For example, E. Fuller Torrey—a prominent new psychiatrist and a leading advocate for involuntary forced psychiatric medications—once remarked that he "would quite happily lose a van Gogh to treat the disease" (1995). Torrey believes that reducing Van Gogh's suffering and potentially averting his suicide would be worth the loss of Van Gogh's artistic, spiritual, and political achievements. For Torrey, there's nothing dogmatic or controlling about his diagnosis. He's just telling the Truth. Van Gogh can get treatment for his disease, or he can be in denial. There are no other options. If Van Gogh causes any trouble for himself or others, the state can force him to accept the Truth about himself: he suffers from manic-depressive illness and must be treated, willing or not.

When Van Gogh's life is approached from a relational theory of the sign, we get the opposite situation. A relational theory sees the diagnosis "manic-depressive" as socially constructed. For a relational theory, the term *manic-depression* does not represent the truth of Van Gogh's life; it represents a relative perspective that is dependent on the interpretive community used to understand Van Gogh's life. Other semiotic communities make other interpretations, and these interpretations make equal sense. Van Gogh may be understood just as well through psychological dynamics or through artistic, spiritual, or political dynamics. The rub for a relational approach is that it provides no criteria through which to make a choice. Within these relative frames, it makes equal sense to pathologize Van Gogh as it does to celebrate him. By what criteria does one choose?

By contrast, pragmatic approaches allow for tolerance and flexibility without falling into the anything-goes paralysis of relativity. When Van Gogh's life is approached from a pragmatic theory of the sign, the terms used to understand Van Gogh's life depend on the semiotic community from which one works. All interpretive communities ground their interpretations in an element of the real, but each does so in very different ways. Compared to reference theories, pragmatic theories give much greater flexibility regarding which semiotic community to choose. But unlike relational theories, pragmatic flexibility does not leave interpreters without criteria for making choices. The pluridimensional consequences of any interpretive choice mean very different outcomes for Van Gogh's life. Which consequences are desired determine which community to join. If a life of talking to psychiatrists and following psychiatric advice sounds best, then a clinical interpretation would be the way to go. If a life of intense creative striving sounds best, then alternative interpretations would be much better. No interpretative community is completely right or completely wrong. All are partially grounded in a pluridimensional world.

Much recent science studies scholarship follows very similar pragmatic insights, and such scholarship may also be understood as drawing from a semiotic-realist ontology and a pluridimensional-consequences epistemology. For example, Donna Haraway uses the term *material-semiotic* to capture her awareness that the "imaginary and the real figure each other in concrete fact" (1997, 2). Much of Haraway's scholarship involves "taking the actual and the figural seriously as [co]constitutive of material-semiotic worlds" (1997, 2). Andrew Pickering uses the word *mangle* in similar ways. For Pickering, science is a mangle, or a "field of emergent human and material agency reciprocally engaged by means of a dialectic of resistance and accommodation" (1993, 559). The material and the human are "mutually and emergently productive of one another" (1993, 567). Pickering uses *mangle* as a noun (to refer to existing cominglings) and as a verb (to refer to the process of creating new cominglings). Using Pickering's terminology, one could argue that psychiatry is a domain that mangles together different kinds of humans. In psychiatry, the material agency that is mangled, through a process of resistance and accommodation, is composed of humans and the psychic life of humans.

Science studies scholar Joseph Rouse also echoes the themes of semiotic realism and pluridimensional consequences through an expanded notion of what he calls "science as practice." For Rouse, scientific practice is more than a representation of the world; it is also a way of interacting with the world. Scientific practice is a dialectic that reconstructs the world and people's relationship to that world (as it redescribes the world). Rouse argues that scientific practices, knowledge-making priorities, and the "facts" they create are not restricted to the laboratory. They rapidly move outside the laboratory to become "habitual practices and skills through which people make themselves into competent, reliable participants in a more or less shared world. Who we are is in significant part who we have made ourselves into through the cultivation of habits of mind and body" (1996, 132).

These approaches to knowledge and the world that show up in science studies and in pragmatic theories of the sign offer a way of thinking outside the referential/relational binary and the polemics of the science wars. Gross and Levitt's polemics point out differences between realism and relativism. But for Gross and Levitt, realism trumps in an uncritical way. They point out the problems of relativism but say nothing about the problems of realism. For them, realism is good, and relativism is bad (muddleheaded and derelict). Such science-wars polemics obscure the risk of dogmatism and intolerance inherent in realism. A pragmatic approach, by contrast, appreciates the problems and the values of *both* realism and relativism. As a result, it offers a third-way alternative for postpsychiatry and a way out of the science wars.

CHAPTER THREE

The New Psychiatry as a Discursive Practice

Having dodged the science wars, postpsychiatry can now fine-tune its theoretical perspective. This chapter takes the next step by considering philosopher Michel Foucault's central concept of "discursive practice." My turn to Foucault might seem odd at this point since I introduced Foucault (and other poststructuralists) in the last chapter as bringing out the radical relativism of Saussure's theory of the sign. But Foucault's insight into the relativism of Saussure does not mean that Foucault was himself a relativist. He was not. Foucault's own theory of discursive practice is very similar to other hybrid theories I've discussed. Theories like Haraway's "material-semiotic," Rouse's "science as practice," Pickering's "mangle," and my own "semiotic realism" all hold in tension both realism and constructivism. They emphasize the role of linguistic structures in organizing human meaning without falling into an anything-goes chaos of relativism. Like these other theories, Foucault's notion of discursive practice includes both the semiotic dimensions of a discourse, which he calls its "communicative" dimensions, and its real effects, which he calls its "capacities."

But Foucault takes this "semiotic-realism"—or "communication-capacity"—perspective much further. He goes beyond theories of the sign to include two additional semiotic dimensions not discussed in Saussure: the "rules of formation" and the "rules of exclusion." In addition, Foucault theorizes the role of what I will call "the human" in discourse formation. Though the theories of the sign discussed in chapter 2 help us understand the inescapable intertwining of the semiotic and the real, they say very little about the human actors involved in creating and propagating a knowledge tradition. Foucault's concepts of "enunciative modalities" and "power" show a way to include human actors in the process.[1]

After working through these critical components of Foucault's theory, I use them to read a central reference text and teaching tool in the new psychiatry: *Introductory Textbook of Psychiatry* (Andreasen and Black 2001). This new psychiatry text is published by the American Psychiatric Association's press and was coauthored by Nancy Andreasen, who is the editor of the leading psychiatry journal, the *American Journal of Psychiatry*. This text is standard on medical school syllabi and therefore shapes the definition of psychiatry for those entering the medical profession.

Foucault's Theory of Discursive Practice

Foucault defines a discourse as a "group of objects, methods, their corpus of propositions considered to be true, the interplay of rules and definitions, or techniques and tools" (1972, 222). For Foucault, a discourse such as medicine or psychiatry, although perhaps seemingly coherent and therefore naturally occurring, does not happen spontaneously or inevitably. Foucault problematizes the notion that discourses are inherent or "anonymous" systems by asking very basic questions: "What, in fact, are medicine, grammar, or political economy?" (1972, 31). Where do the elements of a discourse arise? What creates the conceptual and theoretical structure that holds the elements together? What, in other words, creates the unity of discourses? Contrary to a referential approach that would assume that the unity of discourses originates in the real world, Foucault argues that the closer we look, the less inevitable that unity becomes. The content and theoretical structures of discourse constantly vary from one period to the next, and they constantly vary from one cultural location to the next. In spite of this variability, each discourse uses the "real world" to explain and legitimate its particular formation. For Foucault, the real world alone cannot be the answer.

Once our commonsense notion of the inevitability of discourse is overturned, we need a new way to understand the unity of discourse. Foucault's theory of "discursive practices" answers this need. Foucault's terms *discourse* and *practice* originate with his pragmatic inflection of two related terms from Saussure: *langue* and *parole*. For Saussure, *langue* is the background grid of semiotic distinctions, rules, norms, and expectations that makes particular statements possible and understandable. *Parole* is the particular statement or linguistic production made possible by *langue*. When I make a statement like "Van Gogh is bipolar," I do not make random sounds. I draw on a grid of differentiated signifiers to make meaning. For my statement to be meaningful, my reader and I must draw on a similar linguistic grid. Saussure calls the grid *langue* and the statement *parole*.

Foucault picks up Saussure's basic distinction, using *discourse* similarly to *langue* and *practice* similarly to *parole*. *Discourse* is the background rules, norms, and expectations that make particular *practices* possible and understandable. The phrase *discursive practices* builds on Saussure's work, but it also moves Saussure from a representational idiom of *langue* and *parole* to a pragmatic idiom of *discourse* and *practice*. Foucault's pragmatic move is crucial for three main reasons. First, Foucault's *discourse* is more restricted than Saussure's *langue*. Where *langue* is the universal and ahistorical structure for all languages, discourse is a local historical product created in particular linguistic communities. Foucault's goal is not to address how *langue* shapes all speech. Rather, he unpacks particular semiotic grids to show how they work in particular communities. Second, Foucault's *discourse* is much thicker than Saussure's *langue*. Discourse includes a differential grid of signifiers, but it also includes both additional discursive features and the role of the human. Third, Foucault's *practice* is more expansive than Saussure's *parole*. *Parole* focuses on speech acts, but *practice* goes much further. Practice includes all human actions, not just linguistic speech acts. Thus, the phrase *discursive practices* involves not only representation but also a broad range of human actions that involve real connections with the world—connections that engage, shape, and interact with the world. These connections create a variety of practices that go on to create diverse kinds of being in the world.[2]

DISCURSIVE RULES OF FORMATION & EXCLUSION

After Foucault's pragmatic inflection of Saussure, he goes further by articulating additional semiotic dimensions not discussed by Saussure. Foucault divides these additional semiotic dimensions into the "rules of formation" and the "rules of exclusion." By this distinction, Foucault divides discourse into the said and the not-said. The rules of formation establish those things that can be said, and the rules of exclusion make up the boundaries of the not-said. Together, the rules of formation and exclusion create a tight weave of discursive organization and structure beyond the level of the sign.

Foucault divides the discursive rules of formation into what he calls

1. *objects* (the elemental signs of a discourse),
2. *concepts* (the terms and models in which the objects are formulated), and
3. *strategies* (the themes and theoretical viewpoints that organize the concepts).

Objects are the signs, or basic semiotic elements, of a discourse. These work along the lines established in my discussion of the sign in the last chapter. Concepts are the next layer of abstraction, organizing the objects into larger conceptual models. And strategies put the conceptual models into an even larger theoretical perspective. Together, these rules of formation—*objects, concepts,* and *strategies*—work like overlapping hermeneutic circles that structure the positive features of a discourse. Each rule of formation makes up a part that is organized by the whole of the next-higher level. "Objects" are organized in terms of "concepts" and "concepts" in terms of "strategies."

We can understand these rules of formation—objects, concepts, and strategies—through an analogy with Russian nesting dolls. Objects nest inside concepts, and concepts nest inside strategies. However, Foucault's articulation of three nesting levels does not imply a limit to the levels of a discourse. There can be multiple levels of discourse because these nesting rules of formation may be further broken down or further generalized. Objects can be broken down into even further objects, and strategies can be further abstracted into broader theoretical perspectives. In this way, the nesting rules of objects, concepts, and strategies can overlap with each other to form a series of levels. Together, these levels make up the tightly structured grid that forms a discourse.

In contrast to Foucault's rules of formation, his rules of exclusion mark the semiotic boundaries of a discourse. Not anything can become an object, concept, or strategy. Strict boundaries apply. In detailing his rules of exclusion, Foucault refers to *what is prohibited* and to the oppositions between *reason and folly* and *true and false*. The rules of exclusion are particularly counterintuitive with regard to scientific disciplines—which are considered by many to be the epitome of open inquiry. But Foucault highlights how, even in science, the boundaries of inquiry are very much closed. The rules of exclusion help us articulate this boundary patrol.

The first rule of exclusion, "what is prohibited," is the most obvious. It involves the prohibited objects, concepts, and strategies that are considered out of play in a particular discourse. These topics are taboo in the discourse. The second and third rules of exclusion involve a division and a rejection. Discourse cannot include anything deemed "in folly" or anything considered to be "false." These divisions—between "reason and folly" and "true and false"—form automatic rejections. If a potential discourse contribution falls into folly or is deemed to be false, it will be automatically excluded (Foucault 1972, 216).

These additional semiotic dimensions work to add further nuance to the way a discourse functions. As we learned in the last chapter, the signs (or objects) of a discourse create meaning through a relational grid of signifiers that are pragmatically and simultaneously grounded in the real. But beyond the relational grid of signs, there are many other dimensions of semiotic structure. These rules of formation and exclusion add an even greater sense of inevitability to a discourse. But Foucault does not stop with articulating these additional semiotic dimensions. He goes on to consider the "human" dimensions of discourse as well. Based on Foucault's discussion, I will call the two human dimensions "enunciative modalities" and "power."

ENUNCIATIVE MODALITIES

Foucault argues that (beyond the semiotic) the people involved in a discourse must be considered part of the unity of that discourse. Objects, concepts, and strategies do not magically appear, nor do they propagate all by themselves. They must be enunciated by (1) particular people, who are (2) located in particular institutional positions and (3) making citation from particular artifacts. Inspired by Foucault's work, I call the people, their institutions, and the artifacts they circulate the enunciative modalities of a discourse.

For Foucault, to understand a discourse and to appreciate what causes the objects, concepts, and strategies to appear—"what necessity binds them, and why these and not others"—one must ask first and foremost, *"Who is speaking?"* (1972, 50, italics added):

Who, among the totality of speaking individuals, is accorded the right to use this sort of language? Who is qualified to do so? Who derives from it his own special quality, his prestige, and from whom, in return, does he receive if not the assurance, at least the presumption that what he says is true? . . . Medical statements [for example] cannot come from anybody; their value, efficacy, even their therapeutic powers, and, generally speaking, their existence as medical statements cannot be dissociated from the statutorily defined person who has the right to make them. (1972, 50)

Foucault's addition of the "who" of discourse moves his work from the textual to the human and to the specific people involved in the production of discourse. For Foucault, the who and the not-who of a discourse are central. How a discourse emerges and develops depends very much on the particulars of the people involved.

The earlier quotation also highlights the fact that the "who" of a discourse includes the institutional location of the speakers. Speakers may not speak from anywhere. They must have institutional support and legitimization. Just as speakers are central to a discourse, then, institutions—and the rules, rituals, and hierarchical relations that structure them—are also central to a discourse. Institutional sites like universities, conferences, grand rounds, hospitals, offices, laboratories, and lecture halls all scaffold and solidify a discourse.

Foucault argues that the institutional location of speakers is controlled by the "rarefaction of speaking subjects," "doctrinal adherence," and "social appropriations" (1972, 224–27). By the "rarefaction of speaking subjects," Foucault means that "none may enter into a discourse on a specific subject unless he has satisfied certain conditions or if he is not, from the outset, qualified to do so" (1972, 224–25). The restrictive process of determining speakers occurs through a ritual process of apprenticeship and evaluation that "defines the qualifications required of the speaker . . . ; it lays down gestures to be made, behavior, circumstances and the whole range of signs that must accompany discourse; finally, it lays down the supposed, or imposed significance of the words used" (1972, 225). Those who are so initiated and thus qualified as speaking subjects form a "fellowship of discourse." The function of the fellowship is to preserve and reproduce discourse "in order that it should circulate within a closed community [and] according to strict regulations" (1972, 225).

The notion of "doctrinal adherence" highlights the institutionalized process of producing "books, [their] publishing systems and the personality of the writer [that] occurs within a diffuse yet constraining, 'fellowship of discourse'" (1972, 226). These writings work together to produce a code of belief. Doctrinal adherence to this code "links individuals to certain types of utterance while consequently barring them from all others" (1972, 226). Doctrinal adherence involves both the speaker and the spoken. The speaker must conform to doctrine, and at the same time the doctrine forms through a prior adherence to its requirements. Thus, "doctrine effects a dual subjection, that of speaking subjects to discourse, and that of discourse to the group" (1972, 226).

Foucault's idea of "social appropriations" refers to the fact that discourses do not exist in isolation. They are very much caught up in larger social structures. For example, education into a discourse is not open to everyone, and the distribution of who may and who may not be educated "follows the well-trodden battle-lines of [broader] social conflict" (1972, 227). Thus, education into a discourse is not a neutral internal process but very much a political process of maintaining and integrating the social status and social function of the discourse. These social appropriations must be considered internal to the discourse because they very much affect how the rules of formation and exclusion will play out.

Finally, Foucault's discussion of the artifacts that discourse members use breaks these down into "primary texts" and "secondary texts." Primary texts are "fundamental or creative" texts, and secondary texts are the surrounding texts that "reiterate, comment, or expound" on the primary texts (1972, 220). Primary texts and secondary texts are very much interdependent. Primary texts give the secondary their legitimacy, but in turn, primary texts also get their legitimacy from the secondary texts. A primary text's inclusion in the canon and the acceptance of particular interpretations must be legitimized by being reiterated in a number of secondary texts. Thus, both primary and secondary texts work to produce and constrain a discourse in very specific ways that very much involve the human actors of a discourse. Discourse members use secondary texts to shape and determine a discourse through which texts they allow to enter the canon. Discourse members also shape a discourse through which elements of primary texts they reiterate, comment on, and expound.

Foucault adds that discursive artifacts work not only through their content but also through what he calls the "author-function." For Foucault, the "author-function" constrains and controls discourse, not so much through the individual who writes or gives talks but through the unifying functions discursive practitioners give to that individual (1972, 222). A similar function (which Foucault does not discuss directly) could be called the "publisher-function." Through the "publisher-function," discursive practitioners give unifying power and legitimizing authority to particular publishing houses.

POWER

Beyond these enunciative modalities, the additional human dimension of discourse that Foucault considers at length in his later work is the role of "power." For Foucault, power traverses all the enunciative modalities I've just discussed and is a major force determining the specific features of enunciative modalities. In other words, human enunciative modalities cannot be completely explained by the randomness of accident, the appeal of reason, or the force of nature. Beyond these causes, enunciative modalities form through power relations. Power, then, may be basically defined as a mode of "action upon action" (Foucault 1983, 222). Power is a "way in which certain actions modify other actions" (Foucault 1983, 219). In this definition, power is the force that, when exercised, structures the field such that particular actions are likely to follow. Power is the ability to make things happen in particular ways.

Thus, for Foucault, just as discursive formations are underdetermined by the real world, they are overdetermined by power relations. A new discursive formation is not just a new "systematicity, theoretical form, or something like a paradigm"; it is a whole new "discursive regime" (1980, 113). Accordingly, Foucault argues that knowledge and power must be thought of together. Knowledge is not free from power; rather, knowledge is solidified through power, and power is solidified through knowledge. Indeed, without power there can be no knowledge, and without knowledge there can be no power. As Foucault puts it, "power and knowledge directly imply one another. . . . There is no power relation without the correlative constitution of a field of knowledge" (1995, 27). Power holds the elements of knowledge together, and power is a major determinant of why one discursive formation crystallizes rather than another.

This vision of power and knowledge as codependent and coconstitutive means that Foucault's notion of power is very different from standard notions of power. For one, Foucault's power is not repressive but productive: it generates knowledge, at the same time that knowledge generates power. Second, the power Foucault describes always includes freedom and thus also always includes the seeds of resistance. For Foucault, "the relationship between power and freedom's refusal to submit cannot therefore be separated" (1983, 221). Foucault's theory of power, therefore, is neither optimistic nor pessimistic. Though power overdetermines a discourse, that does not mean that power completely determines a discourse. There is always room to shape, reshape, and resist within discursive formations.

The Application of Discursive Practice to the New Psychiatry

In summary, Foucault's theory of discursive practice explains the unity of human knowledge formations by starting with a pragmatic inflection of Saussure's linguistics. From there, Foucault adds additional semiotic dimensions that he calls the rules of formation and the rules of exclusion. Going further, his theory adds the human dimension of a discourse in the form of enunciative modalities and power. These human dimensions overdetermine the shape of discursive practice. All of these aspects of discursive practice—rules of formation and exclusion, enunciative modalities, and power—create the sense of the spontaneity, unity, and inevitability of a discourse.

To see the relevance of discursive practice for contemporary psychiatry, I apply Foucault's theory to a key discursive example of the new psychiatry: the third edition of a leading psychiatry textbook, *Introductory Textbook of Psychiatry,* by Nancy Andreasen and Donald Black (2001). This best-selling textbook helped crystallize the new psychiatry and currently shapes the education of an emerging generation of scientific psychiatrists. To highlight its discursive structure, I first consider the rules of formation at work in the text.

Curiously, *Introductory Textbook of Psychiatry* begins similarly to how Foucault might begin. Andreasen and Black open with a very basic question: "What is psychiatry?" They do this because they recognize the tremendous diversity and disunity in the term *psychiatry.* They recognize that psychiatry connects with diverse phenomena like "Freud's couch, Jack Nicholson receiving electroconvulsive therapy in *One Flew Over the Cuckoo's Nest,* or Dr. Ruth discussing sexual adjustment on television" (2001, xvii). And they recognize that a typical day for a practicing psychiatrist "may involve [such diverse activities as] prescribing medication to a depressed patient, helping a teenager come to grips with the effect of having an alcoholic parent, and guiding a severely handicapped schizophrenic patient toward receiving needed social services" (2001, xvi).

As Foucault might, Andreasen and Black question the unity of "psychiatry." They want to establish what holds such diversity together. Using

Foucault's terminology, we can say that Andreasen and Black find an answer to their question through the objects, concepts, and strategies of psychiatric discourse. Andreasen and Black point to the *objects* of the new psychiatry in the following quote:

> What is psychiatry? It is the branch of medicine that focuses on the diagnosis and treatment of mental illnesses. Some of these illnesses are very serious, such as schizophrenia, Alzheimer's disease, or the various mood disorders. Others may be less serious, but still very significant, such as adjustment disorders or personality disorders. . . . As a discipline within medicine, the primary purposes of psychiatry are to define and recognize illnesses, to identify methods for treating them, and ultimately to develop methods for discovering their causes and implementing preventive measure. (2001, xvii)

The objects Andreasen and Black point to are *illnesses* and *disorders*. They use these terms interchangeably, and they devote the largest section of their textbook to these psychiatric objects. The section called "Psychiatric Disorders" covers 45 percent of the book's total, and it gives a detailed description of the objects of psychiatry: schizophrenia, the mood disorders, adjustment disorders, personality disorders, sexual and gender identity disorders, eating disorders, and so on (2001, vi–vii). These disorders are the objects of the new psychiatry.

Andreasen and Black signal the conceptual models, or *concepts,* they use when they proudly link psychiatry to medicine. With this linkage, Andreasen and Black signal a "disease model" that organizes the psychiatric disorders. The disease model of medicine, despite years of critique, reduces medical conditions to discrete biological diseases and treatments to specific "magic bullets." Medical disorders under the disease model are circumscribed abnormalities (such as pneumococcal pneumonia) that can be treated with circumscribed interventions (penicillin). Psychiatric disorders similarly become circumscribed abnormalities (such as manic-depressive illness) that can be treated with circumscribed interventions (lithium). Thus, we see that the main concept that organizes the objects of psychiatry for Andreasen and Black is the disease model.

The *strategy* Andreasen and Black use to organize their disease model of psychiatric disorders is "atheoretical science." As I discuss in the first chapter, the new psychiatry paradoxically uses a theoretical strategy of "atheoretical science" to separate itself from the psychoanalytic psychiatry that came before. The new psychiatry calls psychoanalysis "theoretical" to diminish it, because for the new psychiatry *theory* is a derogative term that means little more than guesswork or conjecture. Andreasen and Black join this new-psychiatry chorus when they call psychoanalysis a host of "theories," "speculation," and "hypothesis" (2001, 14). For Andreasen and Black, the developments in neuroscience are so extraordinary that Freud's theoretical methods are no longer necessary. The new psychiatry now strives for a "comprehensive understanding of normal brain function at levels that range from mind to molecule, and to determine how alterations in these normal functions . . . lead to the development of symptoms of mental illnesses (2001, 19). The "strategy" at work here is that of atheoretical science used to create a neurochemical causal theory of mental disorders.

We may say then that the objects of the new psychiatry are the disorders, the leading concept is the disease model, and the leading strategy is atheoretical science. However, this outline of the objects, concepts, and strategies is not the whole story. There is an additional nesting layer of objects that we must consider. Andreasen and Black signal this additional nesting layer when they break down the objects of mental disorders into the further objects of "signs and symptoms." These signs and symptoms are so important for the new psychiatry that Andreasen and Black devote over thirty pages to detailed definitions, descriptions, and categorizations of these additional objects. A listing of this breakdown of signs and symptoms includes the following:

> **delusions** (persecutory delusions, delusions of jealousy, delusions of sin or guilt, grandiose delusions, religious delusions, somatic delusions, ideas and delusions of reference, delusions of being controlled, delusions of mind reading, thought broadcasting/audible thoughts, thought insertion, thought withdrawal), **hallucinations** (auditory hallucinations, voices commenting, voices conversing, somatic or tactile hallucinations, olfactory hallucinations, visual hallucinations), **bizarre or disorganized behavior** (clothing and behavior, social and sexual behavior, aggressive and agitated behavior, ritualistic or stereotyped behavior), **disorganized speech or positive formal thought disorder** (derailment or loose associations, tangentiality, incoherence, word salad or schizophasia, illogicality, circumstantiality, pressure of speech, distractible speech, clanging, catatonic motor behavior {stupor, rigidity, waxy flexibility, excitement, posturing and mannerisms}, alogia, poverty of speech, poverty of

content of speech, blocking, increased latency of response, perseveration), **affective flattening or blunting** (unchanging facial expression, decreased spontaneous movements, paucity of expressive gestures, poor eye contact, affective nonresponsivity, lack of vocal inflections), **inappropriate affect, avolition-apathy** (grooming and hygiene, impersistence at work or school, physical anergia), **anhedonia-asociality** (recreational interests and activities, sexual interest and activity, ability to feel intimacy and closeness, relationships with friends and peers), **attention, social inattentiveness, inattentiveness during mental status testing, manic symptoms** (euphoric mood, increase in activity, racing thoughts/flight of ideas, inflated self-esteem, decreased need for sleep, distractability, poor judgment), **depressive symptoms** (dysphoric mood, change in appetite or weight, insomnia or hypersomnia, psychomotor agitation, psychomotor retardation, loss of interest or pleasure, loss of energy, feelings of worthlessness, diminished ability to think or concentrate, recurrent thoughts of death/suicide, distinct quality of mood, nonreactivity of mood, diurnal variation), **anxiety symptoms** (panic attacks, agoraphobia, social phobia, specific phobia, obsessions, compulsions). (2001, 58–84)

These signs and symptoms are even more elemental than mental disorders, and as such, we may understand them as additional elemental discursive objects of the new psychiatry. The effect of these objects is to shift the nesting of new-psychiatry objects, concepts, and strategies down a notch. In other words, when signs and symptoms are the objects, the previous objects become the new concepts. Thus the disorders (like manic-depressive illness) become concepts that organize the new objects: the signs and symptoms.[3]

Let me turn now from Foucault's "rules of formation" to his "rules of exclusion." For Andreasen and Black, contemporary psychiatric science does not have rules of exclusion because new-psychiatric science is an open inquiry. For Foucault, however, a discourse like the new psychiatry excludes through *what is prohibited* and through boundaries between *reason* and *folly* and the *true* and the *false*. We only have to scratch the surface to see the rules of exclusion at play in the new psychiatry.

Starting with *what is prohibited,* the easiest way to see the inherent limits of Andreasen and Black's new-psychiatry discourse is to compare their text with another. A text from any other psychiatric discourse would do. For starkness of contrast, I have chosen John Mirowsky and Catherine

Ross's *Social Causes of Psychological Distress* (2003). Mirowsky and Ross argue that psychological problems are not simply the result of personal or biological problems. Psychological problems also result from social problems, social inequities, and social injustice in the larger society. If we turn to Mirowsky and Ross's index, we find extensive listings for topics like race, racism, gender, sexism, homophobia, patriarchy, income, inequity, poverty, unemployment, socioeconomic status, and neighborhood disadvantage (2003, 313–20). Amazingly, the only one of these topics listed in Andreasen and Black's index is gender—but even here there is nothing about sexism or patriarchy. Foucault's first rule of exclusion, "what is prohibited," is clearly at play here. The absence in Andreasen and Black's text of social factors obviously relevant to psychological distress can only be understood as a kind of taboo, or as Foucault would put it, a *prohibition*. These social factors are off-limits to the new psychiatry. As such, they can be considered to be prohibited from the discourse.

Foucault's boundary between *reason* and *folly* is (at one and the same time) the most obvious, most subtle, and most pernicious boundary set in psychiatric discourse—with the new psychiatry being the most recent example. The boundary is obvious because the distinction is the very justification for psychiatry's existence. The whole point of psychiatry is to differentiate reason from folly. It is subtle because it is so pervasive that it becomes invisible (as in the quote often attributed to Marshall McLuhan: "I don't know who discovered water, but I'm pretty sure it wasn't a fish"). And finally, it is the most pernicious because it has the most pronounced effects on who is allowed to contribute to the discourse of psychiatry. Foucault argues that those deemed to be in "folly," or "mad," are cut off from legitimate discourse. The mad person's "words are null and void, without truth or significance, [and they are] worthless as evidence" (1972, 216). To be mad is to be out of bounds. The mad person's words do not count. This has been a feature of Western society since the Middle Ages, and it continues to be the defining feature of psychiatry today. The psychiatric clinician, by definition, occupies the position of "reason," and the patient is relegated to the position of "folly." This boundary excludes the "mad" from the discourse about them.

This boundary creates the incredible phenomenon that the patient's perspective is not included in psychiatric discourse until the psychiatric observer processes it. Whatever the patient says may be seen as "folly" because by definition psychiatric patients are in folly. Only the "reasonable" words of clinicians and researchers are included in psychiatric discourse. The result is that whole worlds of possible contributions to psychiatric discourse are excluded. The most important stakeholders (the persons whom the discourse is manifestly designed to assist and affect) are excluded from the outset. To illustrate the extent of this exclusion, consider that, although Andreasen and Black include fifty pages of references in their text, the people experiencing the problems the text "describes" have written none of these references. Even if there were one or two references I missed, it is still Andreasen and Black who have selected these references and not others. The "mad" have no contributing role, and they have no coediting role. To include them would be folly.

Foucault's last rule of exclusion, based on the boundary between the *true* and the *false,* is particularly relevant to the new psychiatry. Foucault argues that new scientific discoveries, "great mutations in science," in addition to whatever new knowledge they bring, also bring "new forms of the will to truth" (1972, 218). He differentiates the "will to truth" from the "will to knowledge." The will to truth desires more than knowledge; it desires unimpeachably True knowledge. The will to truth imposes its exclusionary force on discourse by prescribing "a certain position, a certain viewpoint, and a certain function" (1972, 218). These methodological exclusions limit discursive possibilities by disallowing knowledge not gained through the prescribed method.

Andreasen and Black exercise the will to truth when they make scientific method the only route to legitimate knowledge. By privileging the sciences, particularly the neurosciences, Andreasen and Black create an indirect exclusion that works through sleight of hand. Inquiry is claimed to be open, but it is only open within a narrow range of positions and viewpoints found inside a predefined scientific method. Left out are any forms of knowledge that do not follow this narrow form of scientific method. Thus, the will to truth denies its own desire to exclude all other knowledge and innocently rides on rhetoric of "objective science." This rule of exclusion is a core feature of the new psychiatry because this boundary has been central to the new psychiatry's rise to a dominant position. Through this rule of exclusion, the new psychiatry excludes all other forms of psychiatric knowledge as not being scientific enough and therefore not in the true.

By outlining the new-psychiatry discourse in this way, we see how useful Foucault's theory can be. But up to this point, nothing I've said should be particularly controversial. Although Andreasen and Black do not use Foucault's terminology, I doubt they would object too much to my description of the objects, concepts, and strategies within their text. And although adherents of the new psychiatry would not like the tone of my description of their exclusionary practices, they would likely agree that these exclusions have been made. How could they not? The real controversy between Foucault's perspective and Andreasen and Black's begins when we move to the human dimension of the new psychiatry discourse.

Andreasen, Black, and Foucault would all agree, of course, that there are humans involved in any discursive practice. But they would profoundly disagree on the *role humans played* in the creation of the new psychiatry's rules of formation and exclusion. For Andreasen and Black, human enunciative modalities and power relations play no role in their discourse. Andreasen and Black say nothing about human factors, placing all their explanatory focus on the new psychiatrist's use of science and scientific method. They assume that the scientific strategy of the new psychiatry is necessary and inevitable. Plus, they assume a reference theory of the sign to conclude that the objects and concepts discovered with these scientific strategies come from the real world alone. The specific humans involved played no real role. Any group of humans following the science would have come to the same place.

In Andreasen and Black's chapter devoted to the history of psychiatry, they narrate a story of psychiatric progress along these lines. "Psychiatry," they tell us, starts with the "Dark Ages" of medieval times. It spans the "first era of neuroscience" (which they call the dawn of "scientific psychiatry") and the "development of psychoanalysis" (which they ultimately see as a well-intentioned but badly mistaken wrong turn). Finally, psychiatry culminates in the glorious present, which they call the "second era of neuroscience" (or the new psychiatry) (2001, 3–19). Andreasen and Black conclude from this narrative that once psychiatry got on the track of ever-improved brain science it constantly refined its knowledge of brain dysfunction. The new psychiatry's historical course does not represent an optional pathway. Rather, it represents the march of scientific progress and the hand of inevitability.

By contrast, Foucault argues that the hand of inevitability is not the answer. Since the objects, concepts, and strategies of a discourse like psychiatry are constantly changing, the regularity of these rules of formation must come from something other than the real world itself. For Foucault, psychiatric rules of formation and exclusion do not naturally emerge from the "progress of science." They arise in a complex social negotiation that includes social norms (what a given community will tolerate), professional judgment (expert opinion), and current rules of classification (how well possible additional objects, concepts, and strategies of psychiatry fit in with the existing classificatory schema) (1972, 41). This negotiation process does not exclude the real world from the negotiation. The real world is an important variable in the process, but not the only variable.[4]

To see Foucault's negotiation process in action, consider two examples from *Introductory Textbook of Psychiatry*. The first comes from the change in psychiatric disorders between Andreasen and Black's first two editions (1991, 1995). The 1995 edition contains several "additional topics" that are not present in the 1991 edition. These topics include "sleep disorders, impulse control disorders, and violence" (1995, ix). But what regulates the appearance of these new-psychiatric objects? Is it the discovery of the "real world" through science, or is "science" just the name given to a more complex negotiation process?

Consistent with Andreasen and Black's understanding of the other objects in the text, they explain the new edition's changes by invoking the "growth and development" of psychiatry's "scientific basis." The 1990s, Andreasen and Black remind us, were not declared the "decade of the brain" for nothing:

> Neuroimaging techniques now give us a direct window on the brain, permitting us to see with our own eyes the underlying physiology of mental activities such as remembering, feeling sadness, or making a decision. The psychiatrist who uses these techniques to map the brain is engaged in a voyage of discovery not unlike that of the early explorers who sought a trade route to India and instead discovered America. . . . The chemical systems of the brain are also being remapped, and the mechanisms of drug action in the in vivo intact brain are being discovered. . . . Neuroscience and psychiatry are exploring the last uncharted territory in the human body. It is an incredibly exciting time to work in these fields. (1995, viii)

"All this growth in knowledge," Andreasen and Black claim, "*required*" the appearance of the new-psychiatric objects of sleep disorders, impulse control disorders, and violence.

Andreasen and Black claim that the new psychiatry was only a modest witness to the growth in knowledge—too modest, from Foucault's perspective. Rather than the new psychiatry's development having been forced by the "growth in knowledge" (or the inevitable hand of nature),

Andreasen and Black's giddy analogy between psychiatric science and European colonial exploration is more revealing. I find Andreasen and Black's honest imperialistic excitement about neuroscience expansion a compelling portrayal of the way these new psychiatric objects appeared. Europe did not "discover" and colonize the world simply because of Europe's growth in scientific discoveries and capacities. Colonization was a complex interaction and mangle of what Europeans could do, what they were allowed to do, and what they believed it was in their interests to do. There was nothing inevitable about Europe's imperialism, any more than there is anything inevitable about the addition of violence and impulse control disorders to psychiatric discourse. That these occurred was the result of a mixture of chance, sudden disruptions from the past, struggles among different interest groups, and material possibility.

From a Foucauldian perspective, neuroscience cannot "require" the addition of new-psychiatric objects like "violence" and "impulse control" disorders because these disorders are not discoverable through neuroimaging techniques. One cannot see violence or impulse control disorders on a PET scan without a series of semiotic links between neural images and the behaviors in question. These links are formed through a spiraling interaction between relations of social insistence and social intolerance (bringing violent and impulsive people for psychiatric examination) and professional expert evaluators who finesse the classificatory systems to create a fit. As such, the emergence of new objects in a discourse must be understood in the context of the multiple social relations involved. For Foucault, objects like "violence" and "impulse control" disorders emerge from a complex interaction among the authority of medical decision, judicial decision, the family, the hospital, and the prison: "These are the relations that, operating in psychiatric discourse, have made possible the formation of a whole group of various objects" (1972, 44).

A second example of the difference between Foucault and Andreasen and Black comes from *Introductory Textbook*'s discussion of "signs and symptoms." From where do signs and symptoms arise? Why these objects rather than others? Once again, for Andreasen and Black, signs and symptoms are natural objects that psychiatric observers simply discover through referential correspondence. For Foucault, they are products of psychiatric negotiation. The signs and symptoms are partly in the world, and they are partly created and selected through the new psychiatry's discursive practice.

Andreasen and Black unintentionally give a fascinating demonstration of the negotiation of psychiatric signs and symptoms in their discussion of the clinical interview. They outline several specific interview questions for "eliciting" (their word) the desired signs and symptoms of psychiatric disorders:

Desired signs and symptoms	*Proper questions*
somatic delusions	Is there anything wrong with the way your body is working? Have you noticed any change in your appearance? (2001, 62)
grandiose delusions	Do you have special powers, talents, or abilities? Do you feel you are going to achieve great things? (2001, 61)
thought insertion	Have you felt that thoughts were being put into your head by some outside force? (2001, 63)
bizarre or disorganized behavior or clothing and appearance	Has anyone made comments about the way you look? (2001, 66)
incoherence (word salad or schizophasia)	What do you think about current political issues like the energy crisis? (2001, 69)

The new-psychiatry interview works by prompting patients to give responses in which clinicians can find signs and symptoms. For example, consider the last question: "What do you think about current political issues like the energy crisis?" Andreasen and Black tell us that if the interviewee responds with: "They are destroying too many cattle and oil just to make soap. If we need soap when you can jump into a pool of water, and then when you go to buy your gasoline, my folks always thought they should, get pop but the best thing to get is motor oil, and, money . . . ," the psychiatrist should suspect incoherence (word salad or schizophasia) (2001, 69).

Through these interview questions and the selective listening practices that go with them, we can see how the new psychiatry elicits signs and symptoms. The signs and symptoms are not created out of whole cloth, nor are they simply discovered. The interview is a complex negotiation process that mangles together human and material agencies. The psychiatric questions are not designed to ascertain whether the interviewee has something "wrong with her body" or has "special talents," and they are certainly not concerned with what the interviewee thinks about the "energy crisis." The psychiatrist uses these questions to elicit the objects (or elements) of discourse so that she can put them together into a conceptual grid or schema of psychiatric disorder. The conceptual schema drives the new psychiatrist's questions and her perception of the answers. It selects the signs and symptoms and organizes them into disorders. This overlapping nest of objects and concepts creates the commonsense experience of objectivity for new psychiatrists.

The difference between Foucault's perspective and Andreasen and Black's is that for Foucault human causal features are foregrounded while for Andreasen and Black they are backgrounded. For Foucault, how the negotiation process evolves and how it is propagated depend very much on the particulars of the *enunciative modalities* and *power*. Starting with enunciative modalities, to fully understand how the new psychiatry works, we must have information about who is speaking and from where they speak. As I discuss earlier, the speakers of the new psychiatry exclude those who are the objects of the discourse and those who use methodologies alternative to natural-science methodologies. Thus the speakers are a narrow band of experts trained in a particular way. They are located primarily in academic institutions, government research organizations (like the National Institute of Mental Health), and for-profit research organizations (primarily in the pharmaceutical industry). Increasingly, the funding for new-psychiatry research is supplied or augmented by pharmaceuticals, which means that pharmaceuticals now wield extensive influence over the negotiation process of the new psychiatry.

Foucault's rarefaction of speakers, doctrinal adherence, and social appropriation are all highly relevant to the new psychiatry. Rarefaction of speakers occurs in the new psychiatry through a careful selection process and through the ritual apprenticeships of training, examination, licensing, and board certification. Doctrinal adherence applies to the scientistic-atheoretical approach, and the notion of broader social appropriation is relevant to the relatively privileged status of initiates into and members of psychiatry's fellowship of discourse. These enunciative processes are perpetually reinforced, and they go beyond initial training to include the ongoing role of conferences, journals, advertisements, drug representatives, and so forth.

Following Foucault, we may say that new psychiatry artifacts include primary and secondary texts. The primary text of the new psychiatry has become, as elsewhere in modern science, the empirical research literature. This consists primarily of research journals. The role of secondary texts is to limit and constrain interpretations of research literature. Some examples would include Gerald Maxmen's *New Psychiatry*, which I discuss in the first chapter, and Andreasen and Black's *Introductory Textbook*. These commentaries bring together a collection of research events into a coherent interpretive frame, and they work to reproduce what Foucault calls "repetition and sameness" of interpretation of these events (1972, 222).

Beyond these more formal secondary texts that organize the new psychiatry, most psychiatrists' daily mail includes a barrage of throwaway journals, newsletters, and invitations to special continuing-education conferences. These too may be understood as forms of commentary that create repetition and sameness in psychiatry. Drug companies indirectly sponsor most of these commentaries, and they almost always support the biopsychiatry paradigm that uses drug company products. Drug companies also directly produce an array of commentary in the form of visits from drug company representatives, direct-mail advertisements, trade-journal advertisements, and popular-media advertisements. Clearly, these are also forms of commentary as Foucault understands the term, but they extend beyond what even Foucault imagines in their slickness and production values. Like other commentaries, these various advertising tools work to create a sameness and repetition in the minds of both psychiatrists and their consumers. The generalized message is, "Psychiatrists give you drugs, and that is good."

The author-function for the new psychiatry—again, as in most modern science—applies less to the primary texts and more to the secondary ones. The authority of primary scientific research comes less from the author than from scientific method. In the new psychiatry, this means that the role of the primary "author" is diminished and replaced by research methods and research traditions. However, the author-function is not completely lost; its role tends to shift to secondary texts. Nancy Andreasen's name on the cover of *Introductory Textbook of Psychiatry* or *The Broken Brain* (1984) adds much to the legitimacy of the text. Andreasen's name carries authority, as she has been the editor of the leading psychiatry journal, the *American Journal of Psychiatry*, for the past decade. Discourse practitioners assume Andreasen's coherent identity and individuality, and her name functions as a kind of organizing principle for her texts. The mishmash of material found in *The Broken Brain, Introductory Textbook of Psychiatry,* and (her latest) *Brave New Brain: Conquering Mental Illness in the Era of the Genome* (2003) is thus solidified and strengthened through the presumed coherence and cohesiveness of the name "Nancy Andreasen."

The publisher-function is also significant for the new psychiatry discourse because the American Psychiatric Association Press, as the publishing house of the association itself, is particularly effective in its capacity to constrain and unify psychiatric discourse. The APA Press carries with it a "unifying function" that disparate university and commercial publishers could never achieve. Much of what the APA Press publishes is very friendly to the new psychiatry. For example, both *Introductory Textbook of Psychiatry* and *The Broken Brain* are published by the APA Press. In addition, the APA Press publishes *DSM-IV* and a variety of guidebooks on how to read the manual. The APA Press also publishes multimedia commentaries on categories ranging from anxiety, APA practice guidelines, the history of psychiatry, and reviews of psychiatry, to trauma and violence (see http://www.appi.org/). Clearly the "unifying function" of these APA-published commentaries, each carrying the "APA Press" stamp on its cover, is immense.

Finally, it is crucial too that we situate these new psychiatry enunciative modalities in the context of Foucault's discussion of power. Each of these many processes, from selection of initiates, to apprenticeship and evaluation rituals, to the varieties of primary and secondary text publishing, is open to contest and struggle. Here again there is a tremendous separation between Foucault's approach and Andreasen and Black's. Since Andreasen and Black do not even acknowledge the role of these enunciative modalities in the negotiation process that determines the new psychiatry's discursive formation and exclusion, they are even further away from discussing the role of power in shaping enunciative modalities. For Foucault, the particular people involved in a discourse and the institutions they set up are not just accidents. They emerge from an agonistic contest of strength. Thus, as in discursive practice more generally, power relations are central to understanding the new psychiatry.

The Relevance of Discursive Practice for Postpsychiatry

Foucault's theory of discursive practice, particularly when it is combined with his theory of power, provides an invaluable postpsychiatry tool for understanding how discursive practices like the new psychiatry hold together. And it provides an invaluable tool for understanding how psychiatry's discursive practice might change or evolve over time. My example of the new psychiatry is not meant to imply that other formations of psychiatry, such as psychoanalysis, are not also discursive practices. They are. But highlighting the discursive dimensions of the new psychiatry is particularly important because the new psychiatry is the current dominant psychiatric approach. Plus the new psychiatry rides on such an aggressive logic of scientific inevitability that postpsychiatry must be extremely adept at reading that logic against the grain. Finally, the new psychiatry has become an increasingly problematic discursive formation because of its increasing ties with the pharmaceutical industry and its increasing distance from its primary stakeholders.

But the future of the new psychiatry is open, and Foucault's theoretical tool of discursive practices is anything but a counsel of despair. If one wishes to change or influence a discourse, Foucault's theories do not suggest a Pollyannaish naïveté about the difficulties involved. They allow no facile underestimation of the challenge. But rather than suggesting despair, they are a *call to action* because they forcefully argue that all the players in a discursive practice can have an effect on the eventual outcome of that discursive practice. It is useful here, I think, to take literally the *course* in Foucault's notion of dis*course*. In other words, a dis*course* is never static; it is always en route. The current power dynamics of the new psychiatry are unbalanced in favor of the elite members of the discipline and their pharmaceutical ties—both of which very much benefit from the new psychiatric turn. As a result, the new psychiatric discourse will tend to stay on path or at best to change paths along lines consistent with powerful interests—what we can call the "changing same." However, the route psychiatric discourse ultimately takes cannot fully be determined by those at the top. It will depend on the outcome of various power dynamics involved. The future routes of the new psychiatry can be influenced (admittedly with difficulty) from a variety of positions.

Foucault uses the notion of a "specific intellectual" to reinforce this conclusion. With this articulation, Foucault insists that general or abstract philosophical analysis will be less capable of making a difference in a discourse than will the specific actions and interventions of internal members of the fellowship of a discourse (1980, 126). A key leverage point and intervention available to specific intellectuals in the new psychiatry is challenging the rarefaction of speakers. To take advantage of this leverage point, specific intellectuals must broaden the psychiatric knowledge base. As such, the goal of discourse change in psychiatry is best served by a strategy of recruitment over conversion. Conversion must work by reversing (in individual initiates and in their fellowship community) the whole process of disciplinary limitation and constraint. This is an extremely difficult task, especially because it threatens the social status that initiates gained through their discourse apprenticeship in the first place. By contrast, recruiting new members into a discursive fellowship requires no conversion. Instead, it requires reducing the rarefaction of speakers and opening the boundaries of the discipline. This is also a challenge, but it is easier than conversion.

From a Foucauldian perspective, opening the disciplinary boundaries of a discourse will effectively change its power dynamics because it will simultaneously change the power relations among the members. The result will change the outcome, or the course, of what is known and what is considered to be "in the true" (Foucault 1972, 224).

CHAPTER FOUR

Psychiatry & Postmodern Theory

I discuss in chapter 1 how the tropes of "postmodern theory" and "postmodernism" are central designators of theory in the humanities. The postmodern trope adds much to postpsychiatry because it not only signals critiques of language, discourse, and power (as outlined in the last two chapters) but also puts these critiques in a historical context. Postmodern historicization is particularly helpful for postpsychiatry because psychiatry is a quintessentially modernist project. Psychiatry and modernism arose from a very similar mind-set. Indeed, one is not understandable without the other.

In this chapter I use postmodern historicization to consider aspects of modern psychiatry that have been present since psychiatry's inception and that are relevant to each of the historical shifts and divisions in the field. The new psychiatry I've been discussing is only the most recent historical shift in psychiatry. Though the new psychiatry significantly moves psychiatry from a meaning-based practice to a neuroscience-based practice, the new psychiatry is hardly "new."[1] From a postmodern historical perspective, the new psychiatry compulsively repeats more than it changes. Indeed, using a broader historical sweep, the new psychiatry's shift from a psychoanalytic rhetoric to a neuroscience rhetoric is not so much a change as a hardening and further modernist expansion of the worst aspects of the psychoanalytic science that preceded it.

Thus, postmodern theory helps postpsychiatry articulate the intellectual and historical context common to both the new psychiatry and psychoanalysis. Postmodern theory helps put psychiatric practice as a whole in a wider historical frame and provides key tools for theorizing psychiatry beyond current struggles.

But why should psychiatry be theorized and reimagined? What's wrong with things as they are? After all, in the United States, both medicine and psychiatry have ridden the crest of modernism and enjoyed tremendous expansion and popular support throughout much of the twentieth century. Increasingly, however, this support is evolving into a chorus of criticisms. These criticisms have been well rehearsed in recent years, but briefly, health care practice is rebuked for:

> overspecialization; technicism; overprofessionalism; insensitivity to personal and sociocultural values; too narrow a construal of the doctor's role; too much "curing" rather than "caring"; not enough emphasis on prevention, patient participation, and patient education; too much economic incentive; a "trade school" mentality; overmedicalization of everyday life; inhumane treatment of medical students; overwork by house staff; and deficiencies in verbal and nonverbal communication. (Pelligrino 1979, 9)

This list, first drafted by Edmund Pelligrino over two decades ago, has only grown and proliferated. Everything Pelligrino cites remains true, and more. Pelligrino does not include current "health care crisis" critiques of unsustainable expenditures, gross inequities in access, and huge health disparities based on socioeconomic factors. Nor does Pelligrino's list include the recent biotechnological explosion that threatens to bring a brave new world of genetically and pharmaceutically modified humans. And finally, Pelligrino does not list current public health concerns about the toxic side effects of contemporary scientific medicine—toxic enough, some argue, to make medicine the third-leading cause of death in the United States.[2]

As a specialty of medicine, psychiatry suffers from all of these problems and more. Psychiatry is simultaneously shrinking and expanding in deeply problematic directions. On the one hand, services are being seriously cut. Psychiatric patients are increasingly found struggling in prisons, in shelters, or in the streets, rather than in clinics receiving care. Psychiatrists are having more and more of their procedures denied by insurance cutbacks, psychiatric hospitals are closing, research money is scarce (except for the problematic funds coming from pharmaceuticals), and new trainees are becoming narrower and narrower in their knowledge base and clinical skills. On the other hand, psychiatric expansion is as troubling as psychiatric cutbacks. Psychiatric medicalization and pharmacologization of everyday life (such as medicating mildly depressed adults or inattentive and restless children) are proceeding at an unprecedented and, for many, frightening pace. As a result, adults, children, and the therapists who help them are all being dramatically deskilled in their capacity to resolve relatively minor problems.

Increasingly, psychiatric stakeholders are led to rely on new medications (to the great profit of the pharmaceutical companies), rather than learning ways of working through human problems, suffering, grief, and anxiety. In addition, psychiatry is the only specialty of medicine that has an extensive protest movement organized against it—variously known as the "consumer/survivor movement," "survivors of psychiatry," "madness network," or, my favorite, "mad pride." These activists are united in their sense that psychiatry has been a traumatic force in their lives. From the perspective of these activists, whatever problems they had when they first engaged with psychiatry, their problems were worse after intervention (Morrison 2005).

Yet in spite of these difficulties, psychiatry continues to organize its core knowledge structures with minimal fundamental changes. What are these core organizing themes of psychiatric knowledge? What are the unspoken commitments that have been made, and how are these commitments contributing to psychiatry's current problems? This chapter is about going back to the drawing board and reconsidering fundamental assumptions. There are common themes underlying most, if not all, of the problems outlined earlier. These themes are part of the much larger and more profound context of intellectual and cultural practices within which psychiatry is situated. Rather than focusing on the details of each problem one by one, I argue that we should back up our perspective in order to locate psychiatry in history and, most important, within a particular way of thought.

Psychiatry, as a subspecialty of modern Western medicine, is a paradigmatic modernistic application of Enlightenment aspirations. In fact, psychiatry offers a particularly potent example of the Enlightenment dream of human improvement and perfectibility through the twin goods of science and reason. Yet across the main campus—throughout the arts, humanities, and social sciences—there is an increasing postmodern consensus that modernism is a deeply troubled project and an unfortunate (if not tragic) organizing narrative for human activities. Psychiatry in particular and medicine in general could benefit greatly from an affirmative postmodern critique.[3] Unfortunately, however, because academic medical centers are separated from the main campus by institutional, subcultural, political, and even physical barriers, medical schools and psychiatric training programs have yet to seriously engage postmodern critiques of the Enlightenment. This means that medical and psychiatric institutions have been unable to situate multiple problems in health care and, indeed, the "health care crisis" itself within this larger critique of Western thought.

Of all the medical specialties, psychiatry is the least consistent thematically with scientific methods (in spite of the new psychiatry's recent claims) and the closest in subject matter to the arts and humanities. Because of this, psychiatry will likely be the first to seriously engage with postmodern theory. This book is self-confirming evidence of that claim. Psychiatry (though likely defensive at first) could eventually emerge from an affirmative postmodern critique not only intact but also rejuvenated. Postmodern theory, at its best, provides a liberating effect on modernist practices. It frees them from enslavement to Method and Objectivity, and it allows more humane perspectives and approaches to emerge as valued and respected.

I anticipate that postpsychiatric knowledge and practice would change in several ways through an encounter with postmodern theory. These changes include:

1. a shift in clinical knowledge structures away from their recent exclusive focus on neuroscience and quantitative social science toward the more qualitative approaches of philosophy, literary theory, anthropology, women's studies, Africana studies, cultural studies, disability studies, and the arts;
2. a grounding of clinical activities in the wisdom of practice rather than the "objective truth" of research;
3. a greater emphasis on ethics, politics, and pleasure as guidelines and goals for clinical progress and knowledge production; and
4. increased democratization of all aspects of psychiatric practice (research, education, and treatment).

In the best scenario, the net result will be the emergence of a new postpsychiatry and a new model for medicine that will be both more enjoyable to practice and more connected to the concerns of patients. But before going further, let me back up for a closer look at psychiatric modernism and its postmodern critique.

Psychiatry as a Modernist Project

Modernity refers to modes of intellectual life or organization that "emerged in Europe from about the seventeenth century onwards and which subsequently became more or less worldwide in their influence" (Giddens 1990, 1). The intellectual ideals of modernism are the ideals of the Enlightenment philosophers. Tireless and vociferous apostles for the then-radical Age of Reason, the Enlightenment philosophers advocated that humans not rest with intuitive faith, tradition, or authority but appraise their universe through rational inquiry, natural experience, and planned experiments.

Theorist Jane Flax points out that "perhaps the most succinct and influential statement of Enlightenment beliefs" is in Immanuel Kant's "An Answer to the Question, What Is Enlightenment?" (Flax 1990, 238). In this work, Kant describes and simultaneously prescribes Enlightenment ideals in this way: "Enlightenment is man's release from his self-incurred tutelage. Tutelage is man's inability to make use of his understanding without direction from another. Self-incurred is this tutelage when its cause lies not in lack of reason but in lack of resolution and courage to use it without direction from another. *Sapere aude!* 'Have the courage to use your own reason!'—that is the motto of the Enlightenment" (Kant 1995, 1). Clearly, for Kant, the central focus of the Enlightenment was liberating human reason and experience from the shackles of traditional authority and religious tutelage. For the Enlightenment philosophers, "premodern" life (as I will call it) was rife with superstition and mythical fancy that were holding back human advancement. The Enlightenment dream was that through the liberation of reason and experience, knowledge would progress. With better knowledge would come advancement in human life through better control of the world.

Thus, the principal villains for Enlightenment modernism were religion and myth, and the principal hero (which became the object of a veritable Western love affair) was rational, scientific, and technological understanding. By the late nineteenth and early twentieth centuries, during the time when modern psychiatry was being organized and before the somewhat sobering effect of the two world wars, Enlightenment modernism was in a high gear. Multiple advances in science, technology, and rational planning made it seem as if humans were on the verge of mastering the fundamental order of the universe. Caught up in the zeitgeist of the age, psychiatry was an enthusiastic participant in this modernist romance, and consequently, modern psychiatry eagerly came to valorize the ideals of Enlightenment reason. To make this claim clearer, I consider three prominent philosophic themes of modernism:

1. the quest for objective truth,
2. faith in method, and
3. a telos of progress and emancipation.

These themes of modernism have been prominent in psychiatry since its inception, and they continue to be central for today's "new psychiatry."

THE QUEST FOR OBJECTIVE TRUTH

As a spiritual child of the Enlightenment, psychiatry attempts to "get it right." Psychiatry understands itself as "founded" on the Truth. Thus, for psychiatry, what counts as "good" knowledge is objectively True knowledge. The Enlightenment quest for objective truth rides the same correspondence epistemology and realist ontology I discuss in chapter 2. When psychiatry creates categories like "schizophrenia" or "neurosis," or theories of causality like the "dopamine hypothesis" or the "Oedipal complex," the idea is that these categories and theories represent the way the world is really structured independent of human subjective constructions. Granted, the categories and theories are understood as hypotheses, but they are hypotheses of the way the world "really is." They will change only if there is a better hypothesis. If there are two hypotheses, it is assumed that one will eventually be proved wrong.

Inherent in this quest for objective truth is a belief in *universality*. In order to get something right, there must be a "right" to get. In other words, there can be only one Objective Truth, the Universal Truth. When psychiatry discovers the Truth about a condition, it is assumed to be true across all cultures and across all historical eras. As such, though the category of "schizophrenia" is only one hundred years old, psychiatry assumes the condition has always been a part of human life. Also inherent in the belief in Universal Truth is a belief in the transparency of language. The language of psychiatric discourse is not understood as creating knowledge or perception or even substantially affecting the transmission of knowledge; rather, psychiatric discourse only reflects the world "as it is." Thus, the language of psychiatric categories and knowledge formations is minimized in psychiatric discourse, because language is assumed to be an unproblematic medium for transmitting observed categories and reasoned theories.

FAITH IN METHOD

For psychiatry, as for the Enlightenment, the route to Objective Truth is the "scientific method." True knowledge is knowledge that is obtained through the scientific method. Faith in the scientific method helps psychiatry determine "how to decide" whether knowledge is True—whether it actually matches up with the world rather than being an elaborate product of the researcher's imagination. For psychiatry, as for the Enlightenment, there is minimal emphasis on the usefulness, beauty, ethics, or political value of knowledge. Legitimate knowledge for psychiatry is independent of the context of discovery and is understood to be "value free." As such, the only critical question that can be asked of knowledge becomes: "Is it True?" For the Enlightenment, knowledge is True only if it has been tested against the world through the scientific method. Only knowledge that is "verified" (later watered down to "not falsified") through the scientific method is True knowledge.

In psychiatry, this ideal has had a chilling effect on all nonscience knowledge. At best, forms of psychiatric knowledge coming from nonscientific sources like patient judgment, family opinion, clinical wisdom, case studies, the humanities, social theory, the arts, and so on are seen as hypotheses or conjectures. At worst, forms of psychiatric knowledge not subjected to scientific method are simply dismissed as myth, superstition, or idle speculation. In short, for psychiatric knowledges to be legitimated, they must be tested through scientific method—even if these knowledges are difficult, or even impossible, to operationalize into a testable form. Thus, in psychiatry, as in the Enlightenment, tremendous faith is placed in the scientific method as a route to Objective Truth.

THE TELOS OF PROGRESS & EMANCIPATION

As with the Enlightenment philosophers, psychiatry's overriding justifications for pursuing objective knowledge are progress and emancipation. Modern enlightened thinkers argue that by an ever-improving knowledge of the world, humans will have better control of that world and will be better able to free themselves from the constraints of nature. In psychiatry, "false knowledge" and "myths" about human mental suffering can be abandoned as psychiatry moves toward establishing reliable, value-neutral truths about the objective world of mental illness. True knowledge, obtainable through the scientific method, will progressively accumulate and allow for increasing human liberation.

In psychiatry, this telos of emancipation from mental illness through progress is dramatically operative in the constantly revised new updates in neuropharmacology, new advances in the psychotherapy for resistant depression, and the ever-new revisions of the *Diagnostic and Statistical Manual.* Clearly the goal of psychiatric knowledge, like the goal of the Enlightenment, is progress, and the goal of progress is human emancipation.

These three themes of modernism (the quest for objective truth, faith in method, and a telos of progress and emancipation) provide an unreflected background horizon for psychiatric discourse. To illustrate, let me review an example from a contemporary psychiatric journal, the *Journal of Psychotherapy Practice and Research*. The journal describes itself on its front cover as a "peer-reviewed interdisciplinary journal published quarterly by the American Psychiatric Press, Inc., . . . its aim . . . to *advance* the professional understanding of human behavior and to *enhance* the psychotherapeutic treatment of mental disorders" (italics added). The theme of progress—to "advance" and "enhance"—is clearly prominent even in the journal's self-description. But in a typical review article (with an associate editor of the journal as lead author), all the themes of modernism are elevated to a highly partisan shrill: "During the past 15 years we have made substantial *advances* in our understanding of psychotherapy research and our ability to conduct this research effectively" (Docherty and Streeter 1993, 100, italics added). The authors go on to "review the *progress* in psychotherapy" in order to "provide a useful framework for exploring areas requiring increased attention and research" (1993, 100, italics added). The framework they adopt is proudly "*scientific*." Psychotherapy research, they tell us, needs a "scientific base," a "science of psychopathology," and a "science of psychotherapy."

Prior to the application of scientific method, the authors claim, psychotherapy literature was "shockingly low" in "inter-rater reliability" and could never convince the "skeptical individual that a particular treatment approach has been adequately assessed" (Docherty and Streeter 1993, 100). The lack of scientific method in psychotherapy research created a "demoralizing problem for individuals involved with the effort to develop a science of psychopathology" (1993, 100). In other words, the conclusion with regard to psychotherapy for these new psychiatry authors (trying to outmodernize already modernist psychoanalytic psychiatry) is that without proper faith in Scientific Method, there is no Objective Truth. Without Objective Truth, there is no Progress toward human Emancipation.

A Postmodern Rewrite

Postmodernity may be defined, echoing our definition of modernity, as including modes of intellectual formation or organization that emerged in the West from about the 1950s onward and that have rapidly become influential throughout the humanities and certain social sciences. As

Flax explains, however, postmodern theories are "not a unified and homogeneous field" (1990, 29). Thus, the term *postmodern* can be confusing because it is often used in multiple ways. The three most common usages are:

1. "postmodern art, literature, or architecture"—which refers to creative works showing distinctive breaks from their modernist heritage, such as the pop-art work of Andy Warhol;
2. "postmodern culture"—which refers to the recent explosion in world cultures of mass-media influence, global-village cosmopolitanism, and transnational capitalism and globalization; and
3. "postmodern theory"—which refers primarily to recent Continental "theory" critiques of Enlightenment philosophy and epistemology.

The focus for the rest of this chapter is on the latter because these theoretical versions of postmodernism are pertinent to rethinking the modernist thrust in existing psychiatric formations. Also, they provide additional theoretical background for the new paradigm I am proposing in this book, postpsychiatry.

Theorists and philosophers grouped primarily under this third category, such as Jean-François Lyotard, Roland Barthes, Jacques Derrida, Michel Foucault, Richard Rorty, and Zygmut Bauman, have been particularly adept at undermining the foundations of modernist knowledge. Relying on these theorists to guide us, I argue that an affirmative postmodern rewrite could change the modernist concerns dominant in psychiatry today. Working with (and working through) the themes of modernism already discussed, I suggest that postmodernism shifts toward new, more fruitful, ways of thinking. Postmodern theory shifts and rewrites modernism

1. from a quest for objective truth to a *crisis in representation,*
2. from faith in method to an *incredulity toward metanarratives,* and
3. from a telos of progress and emancipation to a *telos of struggle and compromise.*

By rewriting these themes in a postmodern frame, and taking steps toward working through their psychiatric consequences, I further elucidate my proposal for a new theory-friendly postpsychiatry.

THE QUEST FOR OBJECTIVE TRUTH
BECOMES A CRISIS IN REPRESENTATION

If psychiatrists practiced from within the worldview of a postmodern "crisis in representation," they would be much less obsessed with "getting it right." Psychiatry would understand its knowledges not as universal truths but as useful heuristics, necessarily formulated through the constraints of a nontransparent language and simultaneously essential to the process of inquiry and intelligibility. From a postmodern perspective, psychiatric knowledge (always mediated through nontransparent language) is understood as, to use Derrida's term, *sous rature*, or "under erasure" (Derrida 1974, xiv). To place a word under erasure is to write the word, cross it out, and then print both the word and the deletion. Because the word is necessarily inaccurate, it is crossed out. However, since the word (or some other inaccurate word) is needed for articulation and communication, it is left legible through the cross-out. By "necessarily inaccurate," I refer to an inherent incompleteness and instability in representation. In Lyotard's terms, all representation is necessarily open to figural disruption. As such, words and representations, from within a postmodern "crisis of representation," are as inaccurate as they are necessary. Similarly, psychiatric words and representations are not True; they are at best evocations of the real. Judging these psychiatric words, therefore, becomes a question not only of reference but also of consequences.

For example, consider some particularly consequential psychiatric words and representations: diagnostic categories. As I discuss in chapter 2, to be intelligible, words and representations divide the world through relational divisions. The most basic example in psychiatric diagnostic categories is "mental health" versus "mental illness." Once an initial binary division like this is made, fine-tuning the categories occurs by further dividing the divisions—for example, schizophrenia versus manic depression, unipolar versus bipolar, and melancholia versus dysthymia. These divisions are always to some degree arbitrary and inaccurate, and they always necessarily constrain further meaning-making along the lines of the original divisions. In addition, these distinctions (mental health versus mental illness, etc.) are rarely, if ever, neutral. They exist in a hierarchy of relations. Health versus illness and normal versus abnormal not only work as descriptions but also function as value preferences. These relational hierarchies echo, crystallize, reinforce, and perform other social hierarchies, prejudices, and power relations present in the culture—for example, man versus woman, white versus black, straight versus gay, able versus disabled, and upper class versus lower class. Accordingly, these contextual social distinctions and hierarchies spill over into and become part of the very meaning of the "mental health" versus "mental illness" distinction. Thus, it is not surprising that most psychiatrists ("mentally healthy" by implication) are upper-middle-class white heterosexual males and most patients ("mentally ill" by definition) are not.

I must emphasize again, however, that concepts and categories created through binary divisions are not only inaccurate and constraining; they are *also* evocative and enabling. Though language never mirrors the world, it does partially "invoke rather than present" the world, and it is necessary because there is no possibility of stepping outside of language (Flax 1990, 196). As a result, postmodernists recommend that meaning-making divisions of linguistic terms be understood and used "under erasure." This leaves language users more humble and flexible about the ultimate value and worth of any particular binary division.

Another way to understand the difference between a modern and a postmodern worldview is to highlight the principles of *noncontradiction* and *clarity* in modernism. In a modernist logic, noncontradiction and clarity are necessary for "objective truth," because neither contradictory nor muddled representations can be compared with "the world." Unfortunately, using these principles of clarity and noncontradiction, modernism often limits itself to only one correlative conjunction: "either/or." There is a tendency within Enlightenment thought for the Truth to fall on *either* one side of a binary *or* the other. One is *either* mentally ill *or* mentally healthy. After all, for modernist noncontradictory and clarity-seeking logics there is only one way the world can be. To be "both" mentally ill and mentally healthy, for modernists, would be contradictory and confused. Postmodern logic, however, is less concerned about contradiction and clarity (sometimes maddeningly so), and it embraces the use of multiple correlative conjunctions: instead of recognizing only "either/or," it embraces the use of "and/also" and "neither/nor." As we saw in the Van Gogh discussion in chapter 2, to use a term like "mental illness" under the postmodern logic of erasure and multiple correlative conjunctions is to recognize that while there might be many advantages to organizing the world through this term, there might also be many disadvantages. If so, other organizing concepts should be available for consideration.

Of course, representational terms do not exist in isolation. They are part of a whole network of other terms and human interactions that work together to form a perpetually shifting scaffold for perception, thought, desire, and action. As I discuss in the previous chapter, Foucault highlights the interconnection of representational terms with each other and with human perception, practice, and power relations through his notion of "discursive practice." Lyotard's postmodern philosophy makes a similar move by drawing extensively on Ludwig Wittgenstein's concept of a "language game" (Lyotard 1984, 10). A "language game" for Wittgenstein, like a "discursive practice" for Foucault, is more than a set of linguistic representations; it is a complex amalgam of language, being, and action. Wittgenstein uses the notion of a "game," such as chess or "ring-a-ring-a-roses," to evoke the inseparable mixture of linguistic representation and life activities. Wittgenstein puts it succinctly: a "language game . . . is the whole, consisting of language and the actions into which it is woven" (1958, 5).

The importance of this for my discussion of psychiatric categories is that to change representational terms in psychiatry—say from "mentally ill" to "social critic" or "revolutionary"—is to change language games as well. Each linguistic game sets up and shapes the phenomena it evokes, and it simultaneously guides action with regard to that phenomenal evocation. And each game connects terms and actions through a different set of relations. Thus, to use either a language of "mentally ill" or one of "social rebel" is to play different, and largely incommensurable, games.

Within a postmodern logic, however, clinicians would have no need to limit correlative conjunctions to "either/or" and no need to obsess with "getting it right." Rather, a postmodern perspective would emphasize that mental phenomena, like everything else, are richly complex and pluridimensional. From a postmodern perspective, any linguistic approach, which means any human approach, is enabling and constraining: it simultaneously creates possibilities and closes off alternatives. For postmoderns, a person does not have to be *either* "mentally ill" *or* a "rebel." She can be *both* ("and/also") or *neither* ("neither/nor"), depending on the context and the goals of the linguistic construction.

Let me add, however, that I suspect that even Lyotard, were he still alive, might be uncomfortable with aspects of this last paragraph because it implies the possibility of human choice and agency among language games. For Lyotard, "these are games that we can enter into but not to play them; they are games that make us into their players" (1985, 51). However, to rest with Lyotard's conclusion is to be trapped in the increasingly tired binary between human "agency" and social/linguistic "structure." I see no necessary reason, within a postmodern logic, for adopting an either/or relation to the agency/structure binary. As Lyotard himself points out, circulating multiple language games creates simultaneous multiple subjectivities: "we know therefore that we are ourselves several beings (by 'beings' is meant here proper names that are positioned on the slots of the pragmatics of each of these games)" (1985, 51). Along these lines, in contrast to being forced and played by a single language game into a single subjectivity, recent "postmodern psychoanalysis" has argued that there are degrees of freedom within multiple subjectivities. As a result, one of the goals of therapy can be to increase our autonomy to make choices among these language games that are simultaneously playing us (see, e.g., Benjamin 1998). Clearly, one cannot step out of language, but there is some possibility of stepping over from one language game to another.

FAITH IN METHOD BECOMES AN INCREDULITY TOWARD METANARRATIVES

In a postmodern horizon, where categories and theories are always simultaneously enabling and constraining, there is still the question of "how to decide" among alternative conceptual possibilities. Psychiatry, like modernism more generally, answers this question largely through its metanarrative faith in science and scientific method. Postmodernism, on the other hand, consistently critiques scientific method for attempting or claiming to be a neutral or value-free arbitrator among conceptual worldviews. As Rorty explains, "There are no criteria [including scientific criteria] that we have not created in the course of creating a practice, no standard of rationality that is not an appeal to such a criterion, no rigorous argumentation that is not obedience to our own conventions" (1982, xlii). Lyotard similarly points to an inevitable hermeneutic circularity from which even scientific reasoning cannot escape. In the scientific solution:

> what I say is true because I prove that it is—but what proof is there that my proof is true . . . or more generally "Who decides the conditions of truth?" It is recognized that the conditions of truth, in other words, the rules of the game of science, are immanent in that game, that they can only be established within the bonds of a debate that

is already scientific in nature, and that there is no other proof that the rules are good than the consensus extended to them by the experts. (1984, 24, 29)

Thus, from a postmodern perspective, modernist science itself is a world-view, and "scientific method" functions in a modernist discourse as both a circular hermeneutic "metanarrative" and a condition of truth.

Putting scientific metanarrative thinking in a more general frame, we can say that when a modern or premodern discourse puts faith in a meta-narrative, questions of "how to decide" are answered by applying the Method of the metanarrative. Modern discourse looks to reason and science: What would "reason dictate"? What does "scientific method conclude"? Premodern discourse looks to religious faith: What does the "Bible say"? For both moderns and premoderns, to follow the metanar-rative is to follow the rules of the game. To be outside the rules of the game is to be out of play. Thus (somewhat paradoxically from the per-spective of spatial metaphors), faith in metanarrative functions by creat-ing a foundation for belief. Both moderns and premoderns argue vocif-erously that the foundational metanarrative legitimizes their discourses. However, affirmative postmodern theory undermines these kinds of modernist and premodern foundations. As Lyotard puts it, postmodern discourse is "incredulous toward metanarratives," and as such, postmod-ernism is an antifoundational discourse (1984, xxiv).

Without modernism's rationalistic and scientific foundation, and with-out premodernism's religious foundation, postmodernism must answer questions through a case-by-case *judgment* that considers a complex inter-weaving of *multiple* aspects of knowledge. These aspects include the use-ful, aesthetic, ethical, and political consequences of knowledge (Lyotard 1985, 81). Without a metanarrative court of appeal, different people, or even the same people at different times, will make different judgments by weighing these criteria differently. Thus, for a postmodern psychiatry, the goal of inquiry must not be to insist on consensus but to appreciate divergence (Lyotard 1985, 95). There must be room and appreciation for a diversity of "legitimate" knowledge structures that are decided among differing mixtures of language games and differing consequen-tial aspects of knowledge. Mushy and indefinite, humble and insecure, postmodern knowledge judgments have the advantage over premodern or modern knowledge in that they avoid the hubris and imperialistic control of certainty.

The advantage of humility, however, does not create for postmodernism a new metanarrative trump card. Though there are many advantages to humility and uncertainty, these are not necessarily greater than the advantages of confidence and certainty. Postmodern theory is not utopian. Postmodern discourse itself exists within language and is intelligible through the same linguistic binaries that it attempts to theorize. For example, the terms *certainty* and *humility,* which I have been using to characterize modernism and postmodernism, are also a binary. From a postmodern logic reflexively directed back toward its own discourse, certainty and humility do not exist in an "either/or" relation. Knowledge makers' judgments (sometimes conscious but usually not) to privilege (and therefore choose) "certainty" or "humility" depend on the details of case-by-case situations. In some situations, some people prefer proceeding with certainty. In other situations, the same people may prefer to be humble. For other people, it is best to mix certainty and humility in every situation. Meanwhile, sometimes, or for some people, it is better not to reflect on the distinction at all.

The same flexibility with regard to making distinctions is analogous to the distinction between modernism and postmodernism. Neither has a definitive advantage. In fact, from my perspective, postmodernism does not exclude modernism (or even premodernism). Postmodernism only opens up the possibility of a wider appreciation of the complexities of modernist knowledge. Thus, in a psychiatric context, there can be no external or foundational appeal to postmodernist psychiatry over modernist psychiatry. The only appeal becomes the internal appeal—preference for a psychiatric world that postmodern logics can create and that modernist logics cannot.

THE TELOS OF PROGRESS & EMANCIPATION BECOMES A TELOS OF STRUGGLE & COMPROMISE

The last, and surprisingly most difficult, critique for moderns to accept is the postmodern critique of Progress and Emancipation. I say "surprising" because, in many ways, this critique is the most obvious. The usual modernist indicators of Progress and Emancipation are easily countered by the equally modernist, only opposite, *Regression* and *Restraint.* For example, increased control over nature through technology is countered by increased environmental pollution, increased destruction of world resources, and increased threat of global catastrophe (through nuclear power, biohazards, or deadly new infections). Similarly, increased political freedoms through "rational" governments are countered by increased disciplining of human life by "rational" human institutions like schools, barracks, prisons, assembly lines, business management, and bank payments. And finally, increased liberation from superstition and tutelage is countered by increased sensations of alienation, fragmentation, and purposelessness. In all of these examples, modernist progress has led to modernist regress. Modernism is good for some things, but it is bad for other things. Though this seems obvious, it remains a blind spot for most moderns.

From a postmodern perspective, it is not surprising that the modernist project has brought as much regress as it has progress. Knowledge, and the particular ways of life organized by knowledge, always involve tradeoffs. There cannot be progress without loss, emancipation without constraints. Borrowing from the anthropologic notion of "psychic unity," postmodern theory understands different language games and different ways of life as equally complex (Rorty 1982, 66; Geertz 1973, 19). Each creates meaning in ways that always contain simultaneous gains and losses. Antiutopian in this sense, postmodernism replaces the telos of progress with the telos of struggle and compromise. Humans struggle and compromise with the world—they always make trade-offs between gains and losses of alternative worldviews. And humans struggle and compromise with each other—they always negotiate competing worldviews that are constantly forced on the less powerful by the more powerful.

For example, this "trade-off" dimension of change seems obvious in any fair reading of the new psychiatry's relation to the psychoanalytic psychiatry that came before. The standing joke among psychiatrists is that psychiatry has moved from the "brainless psychiatry" of psychoanalysis to the "mindless psychiatry" of neuroscience and the *DSM-III.* This joke pretty much says it all with regard to a telos of struggle and compromise. The move from one paradigm to the next is not pure progress. The new psychiatry made only a partial progress along the lines of a greater capacity for using neuroscience conceptualizations and social-science operational methods. This increased capacity, though, was a simultaneous loss of capacity (regress). The new psychiatry loses psychoanalytic tools for articulating mental dynamics and therapeutic transferences between helper and helped. Thus, there have been trade-offs and compromises between these different psychiatric language games. Neither side can claim to have the absolute advantage over the other. One has advantages along certain lines, while the other has advantages along alternative lines. Each language game struggles with the world, and the players of one game (who, Lyotard reminds us, are themselves played by the game they have entered) are also in a struggle with the players of the other.

Unfortunately, much of the struggle between psychiatric players is a power struggle that leaves them with little incentive to negotiate. Even if they should desire to negotiate, however, these two sets of players—new psychiatrists and psychoanalysts—would have great difficulty communicating with each other. For better or worse, they work within different language games. Lyotard introduces an important distinction between what he calls a "differend" and a "litigation" to help articulate this phenomenon. He says:

> As distinguished from a litigation, a *differend* would be the case of conflict, between (at least) two parties, that cannot be equitably resolved for lack of a rule of judgment applicable to both arguments. One side's legitimacy does not imply the other's lack of legitimacy. However, applying a single rule of judgment to both in order to settle their differend as though it were merely a litigation would wrong (at least) one of them (and both of them if neither side admits this rule). (1988, xi)

To sharpen this distinction, Lyotard adds the further distinction between a "damage" and a "wrong": "Damages result from an injury which is inflicted upon the rules of genre of discourse but which is reparable according to those rules. A wrong results from the fact that the rules of genre of discourse by which one judges are not those of the judged genre or genres of discourse" (1988, xi). Thus, for Lyotard, "damage" is what occurs in a conflict or clash between two parties that can be litigated and therefore addressed and compensated. Wrongs, on the other hand, which occur in a clash between parties of a differend, must remain mute and uncompensatable because there is no language of litigation between the parties.

Using Lyotard's postmodern terminology in a psychiatric context, in the struggle between brainless psychiatry and mindless psychiatry, the two discourses and their players simultaneously wrong each other. Both have their own criteria of legitimacy, but there is no single rule of judgment applicable to both approaches. Therefore, there is no "court of appeal" for litigating the struggle between psychoanalysis and the new psychiatry. Lyotard argues that the task for differends is not to insist on or force them into a court that is bound to fail one or both sides. Rather, the task is to *witness* the differend and to build structures of tolerance for differends. For Lyotard, differends are not the exception but the rule. We should see them as common, and we should prepare for the plurality they create.

This does not mean that language games never shift or that yesterday's differends cannot become tomorrow's litigants. Incommensurability between language games is not absolute. Compromise is possible, and as I have said, it is a fundamental telos of postmodern logic. However, resolving one differend through a shift in discursive practices frequently creates another differend somewhere else. Thus, compromise and struggle constantly coexist, and there will always be differends in psychiatry that struggle with each other. Rather than fight this phenomenon, Lyotard suggests that we expect it and prepare for it. If psychiatry were to follow this seemingly simple postmodern logic, it would mean that psychiatry must accept multiple and incommensurate forms of practice and knowledge-making. As I argue in the last chapter of this book, that acceptance would result in dramatic changes in the current organization of psychiatric structures.

Postmodern Theory and Postpsychiatry

For me, postmodern theory along these lines is crucial for scaffolding a new paradigm of postpsychiatry. The postmodern theory I have discussed here adds to the theoretical insights of the previous chapters in three vital ways. First, postmodern thinking is critical because of its historicizing thrust. It helps put pragmatic theories of representation and Foucauldian theories of discursive practice in a historical frame. And it offers a historicized understanding of the problematic modernist agenda of current psychiatry.

Second, as I have shown in this chapter, postmodern theory demonstrates the similarities between new psychiatry and psychoanalysis. Although these two psychiatric paradigms are often seen as poles apart, postmodern thinking shows how much these different psychiatric formations share. In particular, it shows the close ties they both have with modernist themes and preoccupations. Both the new psychiatry and psychoanalysis are organized through modernist schemas of a quest for objective truth, a faith in method, and a telos of progress and emancipation.

Finally, and linked to the last point, postmodern theory can help us understand how many of the endemic problems of existing psychiatric formations arise from modernist ways of thinking. Rather than tackle the problems of new psychiatry or psychoanalysis on an individual one-by-one basis, postmodern theory allows a more fundamental critique that grants more radical and overarching solutions to the problems of existing psychiatric formations. Both the new biopsychiatry and psychoanalysis would benefit from an affirmative postmodern shift toward a crisis of representation, incredulity toward metanarratives, and a telos of struggle and compromise.

Postmodern theory, then, joins pragmatic theories of representation and Foucauldian theories of discursive practice and power to form the bedrock of a theorized postpsychiatry. Taken together, these theories provide serious additional scaffolding for the emergence of postpsychiatry. For postpsychiatry to emerge, the humanities theories examined in these first chapters (in all their complexity and nuance) must be understood and worked through. Nothing less will scaffold the change of mind-set needed to get beyond the problems and impasses of current psychiatric thinking.

But theory alone is not enough. Postpsychiatry also needs to begin specific applications of its theorized thinking to current issues and problems in psychiatry. In the next chapter, I describe how this could happen through a postpsychiatric form of cultural studies scholarship. Such a scholarship would provide the tools and settings in which dominant psychiatric practice and knowledge could be questioned and rethought. By forming alliances with the already postdisciplinary and interdisciplinary domain of cultural studies, postpsychiatry scholarship (in the form of cultural studies of psychiatry) could forge all-important connections between psychiatry and the broader campus.

CHAPTER FIVE

Postdisciplinary Coalitions & Alignments

I am immensely gratified when I receive information . . . that [my work]
has contributed to changing therapeutic theory and practice concerning
what I argue are "cultural pathologies" of the body, to helping women
with eating problems reinterpret and revalue their bodies, and to encour-
aging other philosophers to bring the concreteness of the body (as
apposed to an abstract "theory of the body") into their own work.
—Susan Bordo, "Bringing Body to Theory"

Integrating cultural, ethical, and political economy analyses of contemporary popular and professional biomedical cultures is critical to unmasking
links between interests, be they economic or cultural, and policies on
"best practices" for the global medical commons. How medicine serves
humanity in the third millennium may be at least marginally affected by
how anthropology assumes this interdisciplinary analytic project.
—Mary-Jo Delvecchio Good, "The Biotechnicological Embrace"

Developing "Cultural Studies of Psychiatry" as a New Genre

For postpsychiatry to grow and develop, it must build an institutional
infrastructure to effectively bring its theoretical insights into the psychiatric domain. The most obvious place for this institutional support
would be psychiatry itself. However, the current institutional structure in
psychiatry resists this kind of scholarship. As a result, postpsychiatry must
look elsewhere for like-minded coalitions and alignments.

Postpsychiatry's most similar academic colleagues work not in medical schools or psychiatry training programs but in postdisciplinary sites in today's academy. These include women's studies, disability studies, gay and lesbian studies, race studies, postcolonial studies, science studies, cultural studies, media studies, and American studies. Scholars in these fields all tend to be engaged with, or at least informed by, the theoretical work discussed in earlier chapters. From this theoretical standpoint, they understand knowledge production—whether it be about race or gender or ability—as mediated by social and political relations. In general, they seek to articulate these social and political relations and find ways to intervene toward greater political balance. Like the postpsychiatrists I envisage, these postdisciplinary scholars are fully aware of, and engaged with, the impossibility of neutral, "atheoretical" knowledge.

At the present time, scholars in the postdisciplinary domains have had very little direct interaction with scholars in psychiatry, and vice versa. A handful of these postdisciplinary scholars *have*, as I discuss shortly, started to look at psychiatry and psychiatric issues. However, their scholarship is only the beginning. Much needs to be done to forge their work, and similar work to come, into a new scholarly genre—one that I call "cultural studies of psychiatry."[1]

In order to fully question, challenge, and sometimes change the (all too often unchallenged and unquestioned) assumptions of today's psychiatric world, postpsychiatry needs this new scholarly genre to be fully established, recognized, and supported by the academy. In the 1960s and 1970s, the feminist movement was strengthened and solidified by feminist and women's studies in the academy. Postpsychiatry can similarly be bolstered by cultural studies of psychiatry. Such scholarly work and thinking are crucial for the development of a rich, informed, and critical postpsychiatry.

What would cultural studies of psychiatry look like? In its most simple form, cultural studies of psychiatry would read psychiatric "knowledges" against the grain. In other words, such works would not acquiesce to medicine's claim of scientific authority and objectivity. Instead they would expose and examine the social and political relations of psychiatric knowledge production. Importantly, I believe, cultural studies of psychiatry would hold in tension two perspectives: that psychiatric knowledges are real and have real effects on the world, and that they are simultaneously the products of social, cultural, and political relations.

A number of these kinds of study have already been done. Some have been carried out by scholars from the postdisciplinary studies I mentioned earlier. Others have been done by scholars within disciplines such as sociology and anthropology. Some have come from scholars identified loosely with the mad pride movement (see http://www.mind-freedom.org/). A few have come from scholars at the margins of psychiatry itself (see http://www.uea.ac.uk/~wp276/psychiatryanti.htm). For the most part, these cultural studies of psychiatry projects have been done in relative isolation, and most of these scholars are dispersed—geographically and academically—with minimal sense of connection. The mainstream psychiatric community has little awareness of this work. None of it is available in the standard psychiatric curriculum, and there is no dependable keyword available for general library searches.

In what follows, I review some of these works to get a richer sense of what cultural studies of psychiatry look like. By reviewing them as a group, I hope to enact a crucial first step of connecting them and marking them as a collective, emergent genre. The works I review here are important because they lead the way for *future* cultural studies of psychiatry. Indeed, a number of the works I review here have been crucial to my own cultural studies of psychiatry (devoted to Prozac and the *DSM*), which constitute the next two chapters of this book. Furthermore, these works, like those that will hopefully follow in the future, should contribute to the much-needed infrastructure to support and develop postpsychiatry. As I note at the end of this chapter, these cultural studies of psychiatry will aid postpsychiatry in its aim to question, expose, and potentially alter the various knowledges and practices that currently constitute psychiatry today.

Susan Bordo: First Foray into Cultural Studies of Psychiatry

Perhaps the most influential scholar to first apply postdisciplinary theory in the humanities to psychiatric issues was philosopher Susan Bordo.[2] Her 1993 book, *Unbearable Weight: Feminism, Western Culture, and the Body,* was a sustained look at the role of culture and politics in the creation of eating disorders. Bordo used humanities theory—in particular, insights from feminist theory and the philosophy of Michel Foucault—to get outside the disciplinary box of psychiatric science. Relying on this "Foucauldian/feminist framework," Bordo started with the insight that human bodies and cognitive/emotional processes are not fixed across time but are relative to cultural and institutional forms (1993, 28). They are constantly "in the grip" of cultural practices (1993, 140). Bordo used this insight to read against the grain standard Western intellectual approaches for defining and representing psychiatric conditions.

Once outside the standard frame, Bordo argued that psychiatric conditions such as anorexia and bulimia cannot be fully explained either medically or psychologically. These conditions must also be understood as *crystallizations of culture* (1993, 140). Psychiatric conditions like eating disorders cannot be explained using individual or family variables alone. Genetic errors, neurotransmitter imbalances, unconscious conflicts, cognitive distortions, and family dysfunctions are not enough. Psychiatric conditions must also be understood as symptoms of social problems.

Bordo's analysis of eating disorders as "crystallizations of culture" goes much further than the most liberal of clinical "biopsychosocial" formulations. The issue for Bordo is not simply that psychiatric conditions have cultural expression and a social context. They do, of course, but the issue goes beyond cultural expression. For Bordo, "psychopathologies" like eating disorders must not only be culturally contextualized. They must also be understood as symptomatic articulations of deeply problematic cultural tensions and power imbalances. Psychopathologies, far from being anomalies or aberrations, are "characteristic expressions" of the cultural fault lines in which they develop. They signal and crystallize much of what is wrong with the culture of their formation.

In the case of eating disorders, individual medicalized approaches obscure the ubiquitous and thoroughly routine grip that patriarchal culture has had, and continues to have, on the female body. It obscures how commonplace experiences of depreciation, shame, and self-hatred are, and why this situation continues to worsen through the advent of increased cosmetic surgeries and new medical enhancement technologies (Bordo 1993, 66). Bordo argued that the characteristic "symptoms" of eating disorders are as much cultural symptoms as individual ones (1993, 55). She found that the hallmark symptom of eating disorders— "disturbance in size awareness"—was hardly a rare phenomenon. In a study of one hundred women without eating disorders, 95 percent overestimated their body size—on average one-fourth larger than they measured on the scale (1993, 56). Other "underlying pathologies" of so-called individual cases are similarly widespread. For example, the idea that thinness is the route to self-worth and "essential to happiness and wellbeing" is prevalent among women—an accurate description of their experience in patriarchy. Similarly, the notion that "forbidden" foods like cookies can set off a binge also turns out to be common—a characteristic experience of people on diets. Bordo argues compellingly that when a condition affects the majority of a cultural subpopulation, the condition must be seen as "cultural disorder" (1993, 55).

Bordo found four cultural/social problems, or cultural disorders, that she felt were most responsible for this situation: (1) the Western dualist heritage that conceptually splits mind and body, puts a premium on mind, and encourages disregard for and transcendence of the body; (2) the related Western heritage of obsession with control and dominance of nature and the body; (3) the advent of a consumer culture coupled with a disciplinary culture that teaches extremes of consumption and restraint and leaves people unskilled with regard to balancing their hungers and passions; and finally (4) a gender/power dynamic that overlays all the other tensions through "a hierarchical dualism that constructs a dangerous, appetitive, bodily 'female principle' in opposition to a masterful male will" (1993, 212). For Bordo, eating disorders crystallize these cultural pressures through a kind of compromise formation. People with eating disorders both struggle against these pressures and retreat from them at the same time. Eating-disordered coping styles resolve the tensions listed here through a relentless pursuit of thinness that resists the encoding of the feminine as dangerous, appetitive bodies but at the same time colludes with and reproduces the very cultural conditions that it protests (Bordo 1993, 177).

Bordo's social and cultural analysis of eating disorders stays primarily at the macrosocial level. She spends little time looking at the microsocial role of the medical and psychiatric community. Bordo does not give us information about the microsocial politics and struggles within the clinical community that contribute to individualizing and pathologizing clinical frames. She does, however, make it clear that the psychiatric community has much to gain by ignoring cultural problems and staying within the medical model. Should psychiatry move beyond the medical model to incorporate cultural interpretation and criticism, it would undermine its expertise—because these insights imply that eating-disordered clients are themselves quite expert in the cultural dynamics of their problems. And, in addition, it would fundamentally question the presuppositions on which the medical model and much of modern science are built. As Bordo puts it, such a move would suggest that the study of pathology is as much the "proper province of cultural critics" as it is of medical experts (1993, 69).

Contemporary Examples of Cultural Studies of Psychiatry

Bordo's work became part of a wave of critical scholarly studies in the academy that focused on the social and political construction of bodies and medical practice. This work largely goes by the names "body studies" and "cultural studies of medicine" (Price and Shildrick 1999; Lewis 1998). More recently, scholars are following even more directly in Bordo's footsteps to address psychiatry and psychiatric concerns as well. Much of this work, like Bordo's work on eating disorders, starts with a particular psychiatric diagnosis and works its way out to consider the social and political "crystallizations of culture" that contribute to contemporary psychiatric epidemics.

Toby Miller and Marie Claire Leger's study of psychiatry examines the moral panics that surround the social and political construction of attention deficit/hyperactivity disorder (ADHD) (2003). Like many others, Miller and Leger are struck by the intense contemporary lure, particularly in the United States, of using stimulants like Ritalin to turn "at-risk" kids into successful, productive individuals. Miller and Leger define "moral panic" as a "sudden, brief, but seemingly thoroughgoing anxiety or condemnation concerning particular human subjects or practices" (2003, 10). Strikingly, they find hyperactive moral panics on both sides of the ADHD diagnosis. These competing moral panics go in diametrically opposite directions. Many warn that children are being underdiagnosed and undertreated, and many others warn that children are being overmedicalized and overtreated. Which side of the moral panic will "win" depends on the outcome of the deeply divided struggle over the definition and dissemination of ADHD representation.

For Miller and Ledger, both sides of the struggle miss the deeper issues. Both of these moral panics serve to deflect and displace attention away from systematic socioeconomic crises and fissures. Miller and Ledger see this displacement of structural issues through moral panics over ADHD as part of an overall trend toward a "posthuman self"—a self riddled with massive feelings of anxiety stemming from cycles of recession, decline of lifelong employment, environmental despoliation, and redistribution of wealth, all of which are "treated" not through social change but through individualized approaches of "risk management."

Critical psychiatrist Sami Timimi agrees with this perspective and argues that a cultural and postmodern perspective is required to understand contemporary ADHD (2002). Timimi argues there are many factors beyond neuroscience that are dramatically impinging on the psychic life of children. These include a loss of extended family, school pressures, "hyperactive" family lives, and an intensified market-economy value system that overemphasizes individuality, competitiveness, and independence. As Timimi puts it, when you "throw in the profit-dependent pharmaceutical industry and a high-status profession looking for new roles we have the ideal cultural preconditions for the birth and propagation of the ADHD construct" (2004, 8). Worse, the heavy use of medical treatments for childhood difficulties leads parents, teachers, and doctors to disengage from their social responsibility to raise content and well-behaved children. Doctors, in particular, "become symptoms of the cultural disease they purport to cure" (Timimi 2004, 8).

Jackie Orr's work on the recently emergent psychiatric diagnosis of "panic disorder" picks up many of these same themes (2000). For Orr, the individualized experience of floating terror that psychiatrists increasingly "manage" through the diagnosis of panic disorder with agoraphobia (*DSM* code 300.21) or without agoraphobia (code 300.01) must be understood, to use Bordo's term, as a crystallization of culture. Psychiatric diagnoses and increasing prescriptions of antianxiety and antidepressant medications are not ahistorical products of "good science." Individualized experiences of terror, their diagnoses, and their treatments are all coconstituted by the social dynamics of their emergence. Orr does not try to step out of these many dynamics to give a "view from nowhere" reading of contemporary panics. Just the opposite, she uses her own systematic interpellation into these very same "force fields" to offer what she calls a "symptomatic reading" (2000, 154). The result is a highly productive movement back and forth between the phenomenology of a "panicky subject" and the cultural analysis of a "panic theorist." In the best tradition of feminist scholarship, Orr situates her own private stories in public histories.

These histories include state military practices and research methods, contemporary social and economic dynamics, recently exaggerated displacements into a war on terror, and micropolitical and microeconomic trends within psychiatry itself. Orr sees all these histories as a battle over radically changing fields of perception. For Orr, "the battle for the command-control-communication centers of human behavior, emotion, desire, and memory is on" (2000, 172). How that battle is engaged will determine much of our postmillennial future. Will the Decade of the Brain become the Century of the Brain? That depends on what happens next. It depends on how the contemporary political imaginaries and power networks of psychiatry are read, by whom, and how they respond.

Other cultural studies of psychiatry scholars start not with individual diagnoses like ADHD or panic disorder, but with larger developments and trends within institutional psychiatry. These scholars move from these larger trends back in to the details, to consider the way these developments shape psychiatric diagnosis, perception, and ultimately prescription. For example, the cultural studies of psychiatry work by Paula Gardner and Jonathan Metzl begins with the contemporary practices of psychiatric marketing and outreach.

Gardner focuses on the popular discourse on depression by analyzing what she calls "consumer depression literatures" (2003). Examples of this literature include the patient pamphlet *Understanding Major Depression: What You Need to Know*, produced by the National Alliance for Mental Illness, and the popular self-help book *Overcoming Depression: The Definitive Resource for Patients and Families Who Live with Depression and Manic-Depression*, by Demitri Popolos and Janice Popolos. Gardner finds that consumer depression literature almost exclusively presents depression in simplified "soundbites that package a range of emotions (from sadness, to lack of motivation and hopelessness) as severe disease symptoms of a biological depression which, *therefore*, requires a pharmaceutical cures" (2003, 124). This process "twists the scientific process in the name of some other *logic* intent on marketing biopsychiatry and its products" (2003, 127). These oversimplifications are ubiquitous, and they are reinforced on the consumer Web sites of the American Psychiatric Association and the National Institute of Mental Health and reproduced in government documents like the surgeon general's Reports on Mental Illness.[3]

The result is an all-pervading celebration of neuroscience that not only reinforces the interests of biopsychiatry and the pharmaceuticals but also supports an emergent discourse of the "good consumer-citizen." Through the equation "surveillance + treatment = productivity," the consumer literature makes a rigidly repetitive link between self-surveillance for signs of depression, the loss of productivity, and pharmaceutical treatment (Gardner 2003, 126). This emphasis on productivity individualizes contemporary economic pressures and assumes that current levels of productivity are universal norms: "the good consumer-citizen is expected to passively embrace the link between mental health technologies of surveillance and treatment, accept biotechnologies as the solution to productivity lapses, and to leave critique to the policy and science experts" (Gardner 2003, 126).

For this equation to work, consumer depression literature cannot be a thoughtful review of the field of depression research and scholarship. Instead, it must close out contradiction through oversimplified sound bites that prevent consumers from understanding, or worse, acting on, the social conditions of their psychic pain. For Gardner, because so little skepticism exists in the popular discourse on depression, "embracing this scenario seems not only logical, but the reasonable act of the ideal citizen" (2003, 126).

Jonathan Metzl's cultural studies of psychiatry also focus on contemporary psychiatric marketing and outreach (2003a, 2003b). He analyzes the flood of pharmaceutical advertisements published in psychiatric journals during the rise of biopsychiatry. He considers in particular the images of women in these advertisements, and he finds that the new paradigm of biopsychiatry is embedded in some very old gender dynamics. Metzl uses this analysis to highlight the deep cultural similarities between biopsychiatry and psychoanalysis. For Metzl, historian Edward Shorter may be right that "Freud's ideas . . . are now vanishing like the last snows of winter" (Metzl 2003b, 98). But that does not mean there is a complete break between psychoanalysis and biopsychiatry. As Metzl playfully puts it, "the last snows of winter give rise to the first flowers of spring" (2003b, 99).

Metzl's connection between winter and spring for psychoanalysis and biopsychiatry comes through clearly in the images of psychiatric advertisements. Metzl's analysis finds that the products of biopsychiatry actively participate in the same gender dynamics for which feminist scholars have severely critiqued psychoanalysis. The pharmaceutical ads show that biopsychiatry, like psychoanalysis before it, gains meaning and legitimacy through a cultural telos that all too often connects normal to heteronormal. Both psychoanalysis and biopsychiatry work through a logic that pathologizes discomfort with (and resistance to) normal/heteronormal structures as disease. They both posit diseases described as threats to cultural stability in need of treatment. With biopsychiatry, the big difference is that the "diseases are treated with medications instead of talking cures" (Metzl 2003b, 82). However new these medication treatments may be, the gender dynamics of their emergence and circulation have changed little from those of the talking cures that preceded them.

Joseph Dumit's cultural studies of psychiatry focus on a powerful new trend in biopsychiatry research and practice—the use of brain images such as PET scans and nuclear magnetic resonance imaging (NMRI) (2003, 2004). Dumit starts with a basic question: "How have we, as readers who encounter scientific images on a daily basis, come to see brain images as compelling facts about who we are?" (2003, 35). Rather than focus on the "science" of brain imaging alone, Dumit connects the dots between the emergent science and the "virtual community" involved in the creation and dissemination of the science. This virtual community includes institutions and actors that fall into roughly four groups: medical science and systems, popular culture, personal experience, and political economy (Dumit 2004, 12).

Dumit finds that the received science of brain imaging is being increasingly internalized as a basic fact of identity categorization. Powerful images of different brains for different people (e.g., with depression, with schizophrenia, or normal) are taken to be "objective facts," and these "facts" are used to dramatically rework contemporary notions of self-identity. Dumit calls this process "objective self-fashioning" and shows how the persuasive power of brain images has created the necessity of new categories of the human—such as the "depressed human, who is also a type of brain, a depressed brain" (2003, 42). A key feature of this new identity is that people come to understand problematic thoughts and moods as a "disease" that results from neurotransmitter imbalances. The person is not responsible for the imbalance, but the person is responsible for surveying and monitoring their neurotransmitter state. Should their neurotransmitters be out of balance, they are responsible for correcting the imbalance through pharmaceutical manipulation.

Additional work in the cultural studies of psychiatry by T. M. Luhrmann and A. Donald highlights the importance of management practices in the emergence of scientistic psychiatry (Luhrmann 2000; Donald 2001). In Luhrmann's cultural look at psychiatry, she argues that, as influential as research and marketing have been, it was the direct force of specific management practices that tipped the scale. Both Luhrmann and Donald point out that the rapid stabilization of neo-Kraepelinian psychiatry had much to do with the arrival of for-profit managed care. This new player in the psychiatric community furthered biopsychiatry perspectives less by persuasion and more "by *insisting* that actual clinical practice be rationalized in a standardized manner" (Donald 2001, 429). Clinicians were pressured to conform to optimal treatment plans that required the objective methods of biopsychiatry to function. If clinicians refused, they would not be paid. This pervasive "Wal-Martization of American psychiatry" has created a climate of practice where there is little room for anything other than biopsychiatric approaches (Donald 2001, 435).

In many ways, the cultural studies of psychiatry work by Nicolas Rose brings much of the proceeding work together under the broad category of "neurochemical selves" (Rose 2003). Rose argues that the increasing dependence of mainstream psychiatry on commercially produced pharmaceuticals has created a situation where the "modification of thought, mood and conduct by pharmaceutical means becomes more or less routine" (2003, 46). Rose charts the way this routinization of psychopharmaceutical treatments is creating a profound transformation in personhood: "The sense of ourselves as 'psychological' individuals that developed across the twentieth century—beings inhabited by deep internal space shaped by biography and experience, the source of our individuality and the locus of our discontents—is being supplemented or displaced" (2003, 54). In its place, we have the emergence of "neurochemical selves" who understand psychic troubles and desires in terms of the interior organic functioning of the body. Previously, discontents were mapped onto psychological traumas or griefs, but now they are mapped onto the microfunctioning of the brain.

Rose argues that this new style of personhood is simultaneously psychiatric, pharmacologic, and commercial: "Drugs are developed, promoted, tested, licensed and marketed for the treatment of particular diagnostic classifications. Disease, drug, and treatment thus each support one another through an account at the level of molecular neuroscience" (2003, 57). Rose makes clear, however, that neurochemical selves have moved beyond the clinic and beyond "treatment interventions." Emergent neurochemical selves have become increasingly about enhancement. Escaping the binary of normality and pathology, neurochemical selves are increasingly obliged to engage in pharmaceutical interventions to remain competitive in the marketplace of biological capacities. As a result, "the new neurochemical self is flexible and can be reconfigured in a way that blurs the boundaries between cures, normalization and enchantment of capacities" (Rose 2003, 59). For Rose, this newly emergent neurochemical reshaping of personhood is important not just for psychiatry. Indeed, the social and ethical implications for the twenty-first century are profound, because these drugs are reshaping the way people see, interpret, and speak about their inner worlds.

The final cultural studies of psychiatry example I will discuss starts from a very different point of view than these others. Linda Morrison begins not with psychiatry itself but with an increasingly important grass-roots resistance movement against psychiatry. Morrison does an ethnographic study of the consumer/survivor/ex-patient (c/s/x) movement. The cumbersome name of the movement, "c/s/x," refers to the coalitional nature of this group. The members of this group have many differences among them, particularly with regard to whether they totally reject psychiatry (ex-patients), are deeply critical consumers (consumers), or are somewhere in between (survivors). But beyond these differences, they share a basic similarity in that they see psychiatry and the mental health system as more problematic than helpful. Based on their firsthand experiences, they see the mental health system, and the society that spawned it, as a major part of the problem for people with psychic differences and/or psychic suffering. And worse, they often see the mental health system and the society as the direct cause of contemporary psychic pain.

Morrison articulates c/s/x activities as a new social movement. The result of the transition—from the "sick role to social movement"—has been variously labeled "mad liberation," "antipsychiatry," and "mad pride." Whichever label is used, the basic insight is a social and political one. C/s/x members see themselves as part of a broader civil rights trend, and they make several core claims: "1.) psychiatrized individuals must have an authorized voice in their treatment and the system of their care, 2.) they must have access to information and knowledge related to treatment decisions, 3.) they must have protection of their right to freedom from harm, 4.) they must have the power of self-determination, and 5.) they must have access to choice in their treatment and their lives" (Morrison 2003, 79). Since psychiatry does not share these core convictions, the c/s/x movement finds itself in opposition to mainstream psychiatry. The movement struggles with and resists mainstream psychiatry's core individualizing and pathologizing convictions through what Morrison calls "talking back" (2003, 1).

C/s/x members and sympathizers "talk back" to psychiatry both individually and socially. They refuse the passive "patient" role in their individual lives in favor of "resistant identities." From this resistant position, they fight for voice, autonomy, and advocacy within their local systems of care. And at the larger movement level, they participate in multiple grassroots campaigns against psychiatry or for a better psychiatry. The most visible organizations include the National Empowerment Center in Lawrence, Massachusetts (http://www.power2u.org), the National Men-

tal Health Consumers Self-Help Clearinghouse (http://www.mhselfhelp
.org), and the Support Coalition International (SCI) (http://www.mind-
freedom.org). In combination with local groups, these national groups
engage in ongoing campaigns to expose psychiatric abuse, change dra-
conian commitment laws, and counter the toxic effects of pharmaceutical company manipulation of psychiatric treatments (Morrison 2003,
166). Through these campaigns, the c/s/x movement works to change
the mental health system and the larger society. Its members work
toward a world that understands and embraces psychic difference—not
a world that all too often responds with "psychiatric labeling, forced
treatment and dehumanization" (Morrison 2003, 215).

Decoding: The Vital Work of Cultural Studies of Psychiatry

As this brief review of contemporary scholarship shows, there is a growing interest and concern in today's critical intellectual work with psychiatric issues and practices. A new genre of "cultural studies of psychiatry,"
although until now unmarked as a genre, is emerging. But what can such
studies really do? Can they really change or alter how psychiatry is done?
Can they begin to change the beliefs of psychiatrists? Can they affect the
beliefs of the wider population, which is increasingly influenced by psychiatric narratives concerning human behavior and emotions? In short,
can such scholarship really help with the postpsychiatric project?

Certainly the recognition of cultural studies of psychiatry as a legitimate and established genre will help provide an infrastructure for
postpsychiatry. The cultural studies that have already been carried out,
and that will be carried out in the future, will provide a stockpile of alternative and critical readings of psychiatry that can be drawn on by the
postpsychiatric practitioner. Furthermore, postpsychiatry will be
strengthened and supported by these alignments and coalitions with
scholars across campus and in activist groups. In other words, postpsychiatrists will not be alone in their project and will have an array of relevant studies at their fingertips.

However, it might still be questioned whether scholarly work can
affect or change the "real" world. How much impact can such work really
have on psychiatric practices and issues? It might be argued that postpsychiatry ought to spend less time looking at academic studies and more
time working directly with psychiatric researchers, practitioners, and
patients. After all, how can academic words and theories really change

anything? How can they change psychiatry and a culture that increasingly accepts dominant psychiatric models?

These seem legitimate questions. They are also age-old questions that have been levied against critical academic work for years. Cultural studies scholars have often been challenged about the effectiveness of their work. Their studies certainly expose many of the social, political, and economic relations at work in cultural artifacts. But, some ask, can their studies really do anything significant in the real world?

Before we are lured by this seemingly appealing argument, it is worthwhile to look to key cultural studies scholar Stuart Hall and his foundational article "Encoding/Decoding" (1980). Although Hall's article is concerned with the processes of televisual communication and makes no mention of psychiatric discourses, I believe it is extremely useful in showing how critical and alternative "decodings" of psychiatry matter and *can* begin to effect change.

"Encoding/Decoding" focuses on media culture and sets out to broadly characterize the television communicative process (1980, 129). Hall moves beyond the traditional model of the communication process, which, as he points out, "has been criticized for its linearity— sender/message/receiver—for its concentration on the level of message exchange and for the absence of a structured conception of the different moments as a complex structure of relations" (1980, 128). Working instead from the "skeleton of commodity production offered in Marx's *Grundisse* and *Capital*," Hall conceptualizes the communication process

in terms of a structure produced and sustained through the articulation of linked but distinctive moments—production, circulation, distribution/consumption, reproduction. This would be to think of the process as a "complex structure in dominance" sustained through the articulation of connected practices, each of which, however, retains its distinctiveness and has its own specific modality, its own forms and conditions of existence. (1980, 128)

Beyond stressing the distinctiveness yet also the connectedness of the practices within the process of communication, Hall goes on to stress how the objects of these practices are meaning and messages. For the circulation of these objects to take place, they must be constituted within the rules of language, within discourse. It is, according to Hall, in the "discursive form that the circulation of the 'product' takes place" (1980, 128).

From these more general observations about television's communicative process, Hall outlines his model more specifically, highlighting how, in a process analogous to the labor process, messages are "encoded" and "decoded." Television producers, he argues, in order for their product— their messages—to circulate and be consumed, "must yield encoded messages in the form of a meaningful discourse" (1980, 130). Once messages have been encoded, this initiates the linked but differentiated moment of decoding, a moment when the message "can have an 'effect' (however defined), satisfy a 'need' or be put to 'use'" (1980, 130). Hall summarizes: "In a 'determinate' moment the [broadcasting] structures employ a code and yield a message; at another determinate moment the 'message,' via its decoding, issues into the structure of social practices" (1980, 130).

Hall is quick to point out that this encoding/decoding process is not closed. The production of messages by broadcasting structures is mediated and framed by "meanings and ideas"; by "historically defined technical skills"; by "professional skills"; by "institutional knowledge, definitions and assumptions"—in short, by the producer's local practices and technical skills (1980, 129). If the producers are part of the dominant cultural order, they also encode their messages through larger "maps of social reality" through which a society imposes its "classifications of the social and political world" (1980, 134). Decodings and the reception of messages are similarly framed by local and larger social and political structures of understanding (1980, 130).

Importantly, Hall points out that the meaning structures of encoding and decoding, because of their very openness and their interconnectedness with other ideas, meanings, and frames of reference, "may not be the same" and "may not be perfectly symmetrical" (1980, 131). Such a view, he asserts, dispels the "lingering behaviorism which has dogged mass-media research" by shaking up the notion that there is an unproblematic causality and symmetry between the production of messages and their reception (1980, 131). Encoding, according to Hall, cannot determine or guarantee which decoding codes will be employed because the production and consumption of messages may occur in very different contexts and different structures of meaning.

Production, therefore, is not the same as *consumption*. Consumers do not necessarily decode the circulating messages the same way they are produced. Hall postulates some possible decoding positions that reinforce the point that there is no necessary correspondence between encoding and decoding (1980, 136). The first position he postulates is the "dominant-hegemonic position," where the message is decoded "in terms of the reference code in which it has been encoded" (1980, 136). The reader uses the same local and social codes as the producer and thus accepts the preferred meanings of the producers. This creates the illusion of perfectly transparent communication (1980, 136). The second position for decoding is the "negotiated position," which contains a mixture of adaptive and oppositional elements (1980, 137). One version of this hybrid position Hall discusses acknowledges the legitimacy of the hegemonic definitions while, "at a more restricted, situational (situated) level, it makes its own ground rules" (1980, 137). In other words, the reader uses the same larger social codes as the producers but uses alternative local codes. The third and final position that Hall sketches is the "oppositional position." In this position, the reader uses alternative codes in both the local and the larger social context. This mode of decoding resists, demystifies, and challenges dominant codes in a "globally contrary" way (1980, 138).

Although "Encoding/Decoding" stays specifically with the televisual communication process, Hall's notions of encoding and decoding can be used, and indeed have been used, to describe the production and consumption of cultural messages more generally (i.e., beyond just televisual messages) (e.g., du Gay et al. 1997). Hall's work, I believe, usefully captures the mediated way in which the cultural "messages" of psychiatry are encoded and decoded. As I make clear throughout this book, psychiatric "knowledges" are not outside of culture. They, like television, are cultural messages that are produced and consumed within the fray of numerous social, political, and economic relations.

Furthermore, Hall's insights, particularly those concerning decoding, provide an important leverage point for the role of cultural studies, including cultural studies of psychiatry. In general terms, cultural studies can be seen as a kind of oppositional decoding. In other words, cultural studies is the reading, or decoding, of dominant cultural artifacts against the grain to unpack the encoded culture and power dynamics of their production. Such decoding has the potential to change and alter the future production and encoding of cultural artifacts. It is true that cultural studies scholars have little or no access to the production of cultural messages, such as those of psychiatry. However, in their "contrary" or alternative decoding of cultural messages, they can begin to reshape the cultural backdrop in which future producers encode messages. Cultural studies of psychiatry offer alternative readings of psychiatric messages and, therefore, potentially reshape the beliefs and assumptions that will be encoded in future psychiatric messages.

Take Bordo's cultural study of "eating disorders," for example. Before her work was published, the only readily available literature on the subject was produced by mainstream psychiatry. Still today, when people come to study "eating disorders" (out of either interest or necessity), such psychiatric literature tends to dominate. However, when people scratch beyond the surface of "eating disorders" knowledge, they easily find Bordo's work. Her analysis of eating disorders provides alternative critical frames of reference that counterbalance the dominant-hegemonic psychiatric readings. Although her work may not have a *dramatic* effect on reshaping the production and encoding of psychiatric messages, it does begin the vital work of offering up alternatives. Such alternative readings alter the wider cultural consciousness about "eating disorders" and, in time, the consciousness of psychiatric practitioners and researchers who will produce and encode tomorrow's messages about "eating disorders."

For these reasons, cultural studies of psychiatry are, in my opinion, vital and effective. They form a crucial scholarly base for postpsychiatry. In the following two chapters, I do my own cultural studies of two key areas in contemporary psychiatry.

CHAPTER SIX

Decoding DSM

Bad Science,
Bad Rhetoric,
Bad Politics

The 1980 publication of the third edition of the *Diagnostic and Statistical Manual of Mental Disorders* (*DSM-III*) marks a watershed moment in contemporary psychiatry. Shortly after it came out, new psychiatrist Nancy Andreasen called the *DSM-III* a revolutionary book that would lead "to a massive reorganization and modernization of psychiatric diagnosis" (1984, 155). Andreasen's description has become the mantra of contemporary biological psychiatry. As Gerald Maxmen puts it in his book *The New Psychiatry*, "Perhaps more than any other single event, the publication of *DSM-III* demonstrated that American psychiatry had indeed undergone a revolution" (1985, 35). And contemporary historian of psychiatry Edwin Shorter echoes these same themes when he calls *DSM-III* an "event of capital importance" that resulted in the "turning of the page on psychoanalysis" and "a redirection of the discipline toward a scientific course" (1997, 302).

DSM-III sparked this massive reorganization through one major classificatory innovation. It shifted psychiatric diagnosis from vaguely defined and loosely based psychoanalytic descriptions to detailed symptom checklists—each with precise inclusion and exclusion criteria all meant to be "theory neutral." This may sound merely technical, but Andreasen, Maxmen, and Shorter do not exaggerate when they call the cumulative effect revolutionary. No other work has had a greater impact on today's formation of psychiatry. *DSM-III* not only revolutionized diagnosis; it legitimized and scaffolded the new psychiatry's embrace of the disease model (Andreasen 1984). Indeed, through *DSM-III* the new scientific psychiatry solidified its position as the premiere paradigm for psychiatry.

Thus, to understand the cultural and political dynamics of today's psychiatry, we must understand the cultural and political dynamics of *DSM-III.* The best way to initiate this kind of cultural/political inquiry is with an insight from Michel Foucault. When Foucault reflected back on his own work unpacking the historical emergence of psychiatry, medicine, and other human sciences, he had the following epiphany. He realized that the best route (the royal road, if you will) to understanding the political and cultural power dynamics of science and reason is to start with *forms of resistance* (Foucault 1983, 211). By "forms of resistance," Foucault meant emergent counterdiscourses that rise up in struggle against an allegedly neutral discourse. Close study of these forms of resistance has several advantages over what might be called an "armchair" philosophical or critical analysis. Studying forms of resistance avoids the often sterile trap of applying reason against reason. It sidesteps the danger of being stuck in the role of "rationalist" verses "irrationalist." It helps intermingle theory with practice and practice with theory (because studying forms of resistance helps propagate that resistance). And, most important, it works better (Foucault 1983, 210).

Foucault found that forms of resistance work like "chemical catalysts" that can bring to light previously hidden power relations. Analyzing them locates political positions, power methodologies, and points of application: "Rather than analyzing power from the point of view of its internal rationality, [this approach] consists of analyzing power relations through the antagonisms of strategies" (Foucault 1983, 211). As Donna Haraway might put it, forms of resistance help articulate "the social relations of science and technology" (1991, 165). They expose whose point of view is being propagated, whose is being silenced, and they explain why and to what effect.

I find Foucault's insights extremely helpful for understanding and decoding *DSM-III.* Accordingly, rather than directly analyzing *DSM-III,* I will follow Foucault's suggestion to offer a cultural studies analysis of prominent "forms of resistance" to the manual. I focus on Stuart Kirk and Herb Kutchins's academic text *The Selling of* DSM: *The Rhetoric of Sci-*

ence in Psychiatry (1992) and their follow-up popular book *Making Us Crazy:* DSM: *The Psychiatric Bible and the Creation of Mental Disorders* (1997). These two works are now classic critiques of *DSM-III*, and they provide invaluable resources for decoding the manual's many fault lines. In the course of this chapter, I consider Kirk and Kutchins's main arguments, work through key limitations of their work, and augment their analysis with subsequent critical resistance to the manual. This kind of close reading of "forms of resistance" yields tremendous insight into the manual's development, and it answers a basic question for contemporary cultural studies of psychiatry: What's going on with the *DSM?*

Kirk and Kutchins organize the bulk of their resistance to the *DSM-III* around the "diagnostic reliability problem" that they argue the developers of *DSM-III* created, used, and manipulated for their own interests. Kirk and Kutchins put this "reliability problem" in context by examining how the "making and selling of DSM came about" and how a handful of "influential researchers were able to use a historical moment to claim effectively that diagnostic inconsistency was a serious matter" warranting serious attention (1992, 13). Kirk and Kutchins show that the scientific and political context of U.S. psychiatry in the late 1960s and 1970s was particularly ripe for the manual's developers. This was a time of serious "self-doubt" in psychiatry and a time of great "vulnerability to public and scientific criticism" (1992, 13).

Though psychiatry had been embattled before—particularly in the 1950s and the early 1960s, around critical and widely distributed exposés of state asylums as places of inhumane and brutal treatment—these earlier attacks were primarily challenges of psychiatric managerial and administrative practices. These managerial attacks, along with other factors, eventually led to the deinstitutionalization of psychiatric asylums. Deinstitutionalization was a major upheaval in psychiatry, but it did not threaten psychiatry's social foundations. As the 1960s went on, however, several additional attacks arose—attacks that Kirk and Kutchins argue threatened the very foundation of psychiatry's medical and scientific legitimacy.

These additional attacks ranged from the conceptual antipsychiatry critiques of Thomas Szasz's "myth of mental illness" and sociologist Thomas Sheff's "labeling theory" of mental illness to the early historical and political critiques of philosopher Michel Foucault. When these challenges were combined with several high-profile criminal trials (such as that of John Hinckley, in which psychiatrists gave diametrically opposing testimony) and the widely publicized disagreement in the psychiatric community around homosexuality, it created a climate ripe for *DSM* developers to exploit. In Kirk and Kutchins's words:

> These pointed attacks constituted a much more fundamental attack on psychiatry than criticisms of clinical effectiveness or its hospitals. Services can always be improved, access to them for the poor arranged, and patients' rights protected. On the other hand, if mental illness does not exist, if psychiatric symptoms have little to do with medical science, if the entire mental health enterprise is a carefully structured fiction about life's normal troubles, and if psychiatrists are policemen in white coats, then psychiatry confronts a much more serious problem. (1992, 22)

Kirk and Kutchins argue that these attacks effectively challenged the conceptual integrity of psychiatry as an enterprise and left many psychiatrists feeling that psychiatry itself was in critical condition.

It was in this embattled context that the problem of "diagnostic reliability" took on major proportions within psychiatry. But how, exactly, did this come about? As it happened, simultaneous with these external attacks, psychiatry was embarking on an internal project of revising older forms of its diagnostic manual. Diagnostic revision had happened in the past, but this particular revision of the manual was to change greatly the fortunes of *DSM*. Through the 1960s, *DSM* served a minimal role in psychiatry. The two earlier editions of the *Diagnostic and Statistical Manual,* *DSM-I* (1952) and *DSM-II* (1968), were small documents with brief descriptions of diagnostic categories. They served largely documentary and administrative purposes. After the 1968 revision, however, there was a push for a major overhaul and a call for a much more extensive manual. Kirk and Kutchins argue that the push for change drew momentum from psychiatry's insecurities and vulnerabilities.

A key feature of this argument centers on how the *DSM-III* developers transformed psychiatry's multiple conceptual and political problems into a new form and a new problem: *the reliability problem. DSM-III* developers claimed that "without diagnostic reliability" no further progress could be made in psychiatry and psychiatry could not stand up to its critics. Thus, *DSM-III* developers transformed the reliability problem into the key "symbol of the profession's self-doubts" (Kirk and Kutchins 1992, 13). In addition, *DSM-III* developers translated the reliability problem into a technical problem that they promised to solve through complex social-science research methodology. They used these social-science research methods to demonstrate that prior psychiatric reliability was unacceptable, that more complex criteria of evaluation and measures of agreement were needed, and that only those investigators with sophisticated research backgrounds could be expected to solve psychiatry's dire reliability problem.

As a result of this process, psychiatry's thick conceptual and political problems (critiques of which were gaining momentum from several quarters) were rearticulated into the thin, but all-consuming, technical problem of reliability. Kirk and Kutchins point to two advantages of transforming psychiatry's problems into technical-reliability problems:

> The first was that [they] appeared to be more solvable than prob-lems of validity, at least in controlled research settings. The second advantage, an unintended by-product of many scientific advances [like *DSM-III*], was that the technical solutions proposed and the gauge developed to measure their success were beyond the easy comprehension of clinicians and public alike. (1992, 35)

The first advantage was a general one that applied to psychiatry as a pro-fession. The other was an advantage for psychiatric researchers as a sub-set of the profession. The reliability problem effectively effaced the legit-imacy debate about psychiatry as a whole. It turned deep public misgivings about psychiatry into private laboratory investigations of tech-nical psychiatric research questions. In addition, the reliability problem deskilled clinical assessments of mental diagnostic categories and legiti-mated a new form of diagnostic expert: the research psychiatrist.

Clearly, the reliability problem guaranteed a prominent role in psy-chiatry for diagnostic researchers. Kirk and Kutchins explain that "the [reliability] problem was embedded in a closely knit research commu-nity, which accepted responsibility for solving the problem, on its own terms and in its own territory" (1992, 44). *DSM-III* developers created a world in which the mysteries of psychiatry, once transferred into narrow questions of reliability, were to be solved by superior techniques, rigor-ous control, and the right kind of training. This placed research psychi-atrists center stage. By emphasizing the allegedly sorry state of psychi-atric reliability in the past and claiming they could do better, diagnostic research psychiatrists made a place for themselves at the top of the psy-chiatric hierarchy. In Kirk and Kutchins's words, these psychiatrists effectively undermined the objections of their opponents, particularly psychotherapists with a Freudian orientation, who constituted the majority of the APA. The eventual coup, led by psychiatric researchers, successfully used the language, paradigms, and technology of research to gain influence over clinical language and practice. Thus, *DSM-III* was presented not only as a solution to the problem of psychiatric reliability, but as the embodiment of a new science of psychiatry. (1992, 14)

With great political savvy, diagnostic research psychiatrists used the reliability problem to transform psychiatry and to place themselves at the top of the psychiatric heap.

Bad Science

But as Kirk and Kutchins make clear, *DSM-III* developers accomplished this most remarkable transformation of psychiatry through manipulation and distortion of key research findings. Kirk and Kutchins critically examine the developers' repeated claims that the manual was a tremendous scientific improvement over older methods. They focus on the field trials of the manual's diagnostic system, which constituted the linchpin of the developers' evidence for having improved diagnostic reliability. Kirk and Kutchins's reanalysis of this data concludes that "even using the modest standards [of improvement] suggested by the developers, we find that the studies so frequently cited to claim success in resolving the reliability problem were flawed, incompletely reported, and inconsistent" (1992, 15). Despite all the hype of the new manual, Kirk and Kutchins convincingly show that *DSM-III* developers gave misleading interpretations of their field-trial data, interpretations that greatly exaggerated the new manual's success.

In their reanalysis of the field-trial data, Kirk and Kutchins start with a straightforward question: "Was the new diagnostic reliability as clear and convincing as it was described by the proponents of DSM-III?" (1992, 141). They use this question to go back to the reliability data and ask, in effect, "Where's the beef?" *DSM-III* developers said that they had improved diagnostic reliability; what is the empirical evidence for that claim? Kirk and Kutchins find no beef and no empirical evidence. Instead, they find a "gross inconsistency between the answers offered by the developers and the empirical facts" (1992, 141). Rather than a balanced report of the results, *DSM* developers use a "language which is all positive. Even in the text where they acknowledge [equivocal data], the authors quickly obscure them in a tide of good news" (1992, 74). The developers frequently use evaluative terms like "very high, quite satisfactory, and amazingly high" in a grossly misleading fashion in order to vastly inflate the results of their field trials, and they contrast these misleading interpretations with more "accurate summaries" of data that could have been given (Kirk and Kutchins 1992, 74, 66). In short, the scientific evidence for *DSM-III* does not support the dramatic and bold claims of its developers.

Kirk and Kutchins consider their work to be a rhetorical critique of *DSM-III* because they find the scientific facts of the manual to be rhetorically distorted. But I believe it would be much better to see their work as a straightforward "scientific critique." If we put Kirk and Kutchins's work in the terms used by philosopher of science Sandra Harding, we see that their method primarily involves close empirical analysis of the facts. They do not step back to consider the broader rhetorical frames for the collection and interpretation of these facts. In Harding's terms, Kirk and Kutchins accuse *DSM-III* developers of "bad science" (Harding 1986, 25) because the developers distorted and manipulated their data. They misused their power, and they irresponsibly promoted the self-interests of psychiatrists and researchers. By doing this, *DSM-III* developers violated the internal principles of good science.

Going further, Kirk and Kutchins's implicit solution for the developers' "bad science" is more (and better) science. Harding would characterize Kirk and Kutchins's solution to the problem as follows: "if scientists would just follow more rigorously and carefully the existing methods and norms of research," any bias in scientific knowledge would correct itself (Harding 1993, 51). That is just what Kirk and Kutchins do in *The Selling of* DSM. By more rigorously reviewing the field trials, they correct for the bias of self-interest in the *DSM* developers' reports.

Conceptualizing Kirk and Kutchins's critique of *DSM-III* as a "bad-science" rather than a "rhetorical" critique allows us to better see how Kirk and Kutchins's work fits with other critiques of *DSM-III*. In making a bad-science critique, Kirk and Kutchins join a host of other authors who criticize the scientific details of the *DSM-III*. There has been no shortage of these kinds of critiques of the manual. Diagnostic research psychiatrist Allen Frances once described the scientific critiques of *DSM* as running along a gamut from "A to Z":

Relation of Axis I to Axis II
Biological and psychological test results
Categories versus dimensions
Diagnosis versus definition
Education
Field trials
Generalizability
Hierarchies
Illness versus syndrome
Judgment
Kultur
Lumping or splitting
Mental disorder
New diagnoses
Openness
Prototypes
Quality control
Rates of prevalence and incidence
Subthreshold conditions
Theoretical neutrality
Users
Validation
When
Xenophilia versus xenophobia
Yonder
Zeal (Frances et al. 1991)

These scientific critiques of the *DSM* have come both from both inside and outside the *DSM* developer community, and they present no lightweight problems for the manual. The most devastating of these critiques comes under *V*, for *Validation*. The validity critique of the manual has been so strong that *DSM* science scholars (both insiders and outsiders) express serious doubts as to whether there is any meaningful connection between the diagnoses of the *DSM* and the "real world" of human mental suffering (Cooksey and Brown 1998; Kupfer, First, and Regier 2002).

When all the scientific problems are taken together, they can leave reviewers wondering if there is any scientific merit to the manual at all. Indeed, senior psychologist Arthur Houts has reached that very conclusion: "after 25 years of following changes in the various editions of the

DSMs, I have concluded that there is far more pseudoscience than real science in the modern DSMs" (2002, 17).

But surprisingly, even though bad-science critiques can be quiet harsh, *DSM* developers do not generally discourage this kind of critique. As long as *DSM* critiques are couched in "bad-science" language, *DSM* developers are open and even welcoming to these kinds of critiques and debates. They use them to legitimize perpetual funding for *DSM* research and to justify continued "new and improved" versions of the manual—such as the revised *DSM-III-R* (published in 1987), the follow-up *DSM-IV* (published in 1994), and the planned *DSM-V* (projected to be out in 2010). So far, the actual changes to the manual resulting from these "bad-science" critiques have been relatively minimal. Both the *DSM-III-R* and the *DSM-IV* largely carried over the innovations of the first *DSM-III*. But the situation does not have to stay this way. Bad-science critiques can, at least in principle, lead to major overhauls. Indeed, the kind of tinkering that characterized the *DSM-III-R* and *DSM-IV* may very well stop with the next edition. The *DSM-V* developers, by all indications, have much more ambitious overhaul plans in mind (Kupfer, First, and Regier 2002).

It is important to emphasize, however, that even though *DSM-III/IV/V* developers have been open to "bad-science" critiques, they have not been open to deeper critiques that question the basic research traditions and assumptions of the manual. For example, the developers have not been open to robust "rhetorical" critique that seriously questions the core rhetorical frames of the manual. Kirk and Kutchins unfortunately do not make this deeper level of rhetorical critique, but their efforts do provide the resources needed to take us in that direction.

Bad Rhetoric

Even though the subtitle of Kirk and Kutchins's book is *The Rhetoric of Science in Psychiatry*, they do not sufficiently consider the role of "rhetorical language" in the *DSM-III* developers' methods. Kirk and Kutchins fail to make this move because *rhetoric* for them means something external to the facts: an embellishment or perhaps a commentary on scientific data, rather than something integral to the data itself. Kirk and Kutchins base their "rhetorical critique" on a bright-line distinction between the "facts" of *DSM-III* field trials and the "rhetoric" used to describe these facts. By keeping this distinction intact, they are able to argue that *DSM* developers rhetorically exaggerated the facts of the manual. But the distinction hurts Kirk and Kutchins as much as it helps them. It prevents them from stepping back from the details to see how the *DSM-III* developers' rhetorical frame significantly affected the facts the developers "discovered." And furthermore, it prevents them from recognizing that alternative rhetorical frames would have produced alternative facts.

Kirk and Kutchins's basic assumptions regarding the relations between "facts" and "rhetoric" have a long heritage in the Western tradition, traceable at least to the ancient Greek distinction between philosophy (love of knowledge) and rhetoric (the craft of persuasion). But there is another way to consider the fact/rhetoric distinction. Recent work in rhetorical theory has built extensively on the implications of the emergence of "theory" across the humanities (Gaonkar 1990). The key conclusion from this recent work—which Barry Brummett calls "postmodern rhetoric" and John Nelson and Allan Megill call the "rhetoric of inquiry"—is that the relation between "rhetoric" and "facts" (or "rhetoric" and "truth") is better seen as intertwined than as extrinsic (Brummett 1999; J. Nelson, Megill, and McCloskey 1987).[1]

If Kirk and Kutchins had followed this work in rhetorical theory and blurred the fact/rhetoric distinction, they would have been in a better position to critique the rhetorical frames of *DSM-III* research. The critique of rhetorical frames goes beyond an internal bad-science critique and introduces what Harding calls a "science as usual" critique (1991, 58). Science-as-usual critiques open up questions about the very assumptions of science. They highlight the way dominant scientific discourses do not develop neutral methodological models, distinctions, and priorities outside of a field of power and only later hold to these methodological styles with the tenacity characteristic of a battle. The models, distinctions, and priorities themselves are part of the power struggle between dominant and alternative approaches.

Science-as-usual critiques introduce deeper rhetorical questions than Kirk and Kutchins are able to ask. For example, what rhetorical tradition is being followed in pursuit of "the facts"? How is that rhetorical tradition used to perceive, organize, manipulate, and interpret the data? And what are the effects of choosing one tradition over another? As Brummett makes clear in his work on postmodern rhetoric, rhetorical choices are always "double" choices. On the one hand, they represent choices about the "reality" they advocate, and on the other hand, they represent unspoken choices about the proper "methods," or research traditions, for reaching and legitimizing that reality (Brummett 1999, 166).

Expanding Kirk and Kutchins's work to introduce a deeper rhetorical critique of the *DSM* involves teasing out the rhetorical frame of the current manual and comparing that frame with alternative rhetorical options. The best way to do this is to connect a rhetorical discussion of *DSM* with the literature on "models of madness." Models of madness operate very much like a rhetorical frame: they work as an underlying organizing structure that guides the perception, selection, and methodological manipulation of psychic data. Models of madness frame and select certain aspects of a perceived human reality and make them more salient than others. Each model promotes its own problem definitions, explanatory concepts, research methods, and treatment recommendations.[2]

Though the *DSM-III* developers claim to use a neutral rhetorical frame, when we connect their work with the models-of-madness literature, we see that they actually use a very rigid "disease model" (also called the "medical model"). The central tenets of the disease model include the following:

- Mental pathology is accompanied by physical pathology
- Mental illness can be classified as distinct disorders that have characteristic common features
- Mental illness is biologically disadvantageous and handicapping
- The causes of mental pathology are explicable in terms of physical illness (Tyrer and Steinberg 1998, 10)

The disease model in psychiatry forces psychiatric observation and research to emphasize signs, symptoms, formal mental-status exams, lab tests, differential diagnosis, pathophysiology, etiology, medical treatments, and prognosis.

The larger rhetorical frame for the disease model is based on natural-science frames of objectivity, precision, and reliability. As philosopher Charles Taylor points out, there has been a long tradition in social science of trying to understand humans through the methods of natural science. Taylor explains that because the natural sciences have been so seemingly successful at explaining the natural world, "the temptation has been overwhelming to reconstruct the sciences of man on the same model" (1977, 105). But a host of philosophers have pointed out the problems with this approach. Human experience, human choice, and human action are sufficiently different from the inanimate physical domain that there exists an unbridgeable gap between human studies and the natural sciences. Humans may be made of physical material, but attempts to study humans with natural-science methods alone turn out to be ludicrously arid and incomplete (Lewis 1994).[3]

Despite these serious philosophical reservations, *DSM-III* developers fall straight into the temptations of natural science. With their unbridled enthusiasm for the disease model, *DSM-III* developers wholeheartedly embrace a natural-science rhetorical frame for psychiatric research. This embrace of natural science means there was nothing "neutral" about the frame for *DSM-III*. The manual highlights, prioritizes, and organizes the "facts" of mental illness to suit the particular frame of the disease model. From the time of its publication forward, the disease model legitimized by *DSM-III* has become so dominant that it may seem that there are no alternative models for psychic diagnosis. But that is hardly the case. There is a wealth of treatment varieties for psychic distress. R. Corsini and D. Wedding's *Current Psychotherapies* (1995) lists over four hundred different systems of psychic treatments, and it only scratches the surface. Each treatment variety has its own way of assessing what is wrong and applying that assessment to treatment interventions. Each treatment, in effect, has its own unique rhetorical frame for diagnosis.

Thus, a deeper rhetorical critique of the *DSM* must ask: Why choose one particular rhetorical frame for the manual and disregard all others? Rather than a natural-science frame, why not choose a phenomenological frame? Why not a feminist frame, or a disability studies frame, or a gay and lesbian frame, or a Buddhist frame? Indeed, why must there a single frame and a single diagnostic system? Why not multiple models of diagnosis based on multiple models of madness? In sharp contrast to the natural-science approach of *DSM-III* developers, postmodern rhetorical theory would not hide rhetorical frames through sleight of hand (like claiming to be theory neutral), nor would it close out alternative rhetorical frames in favor of a single frame. Many models of madness can be applied to psychic distress, and no one model is right. They all have advantages and disadvantages. In the end, the choice of model or frame depends not on science but on the perspectives and values of the person and persons involved.

Though a detailed comparative analysis of the models is beyond the scope of this chapter, the details are not necessary to make this very basic rhetorical claim: *DSM-III* developers ushered in an approach to psychic diagnosis that is not only bad science but also bad rhetoric. To make this argument good, all I need to show is that for many stakeholders in psychiatry the advantages of the disease model do not exceed its disadvantages. The main advantages claimed for the disease model are improved diagnostic reliability, clarity, and promotion of differential diagnosis (Andreasen and Black 2001, 34–35). It is also fair to say that natural-science models like *DSM-III* have advantages in researching and treating the most clearly physical dimensions of the human psyche: bodies, brains, neurotransmitters. As such, natural-science models will have advantages in developing biological models of psychiatric illness and creating pharmacologic and other somatic treatment interventions.

But beyond these advantages, there are also many disadvantages to the *DSM-III* disease-model approach. Indeed, most critics of contemporary psychiatry focus their critiques on problems with the disease model. These critiques are many, and the problems with disease-model psychiatry are severe. The rhetorical frame of the disease model tends to

- naturalize and reify "mental illness";
- feed into the medicalization of deviance;
- feed into psychiatry as an agent of normalization, state control, and multicultural oppression;
- feed into the pharmaceutical industry boondoggle; and
- rest on a natural-science model approach to humans that excludes other approaches and excludes multiple approaches.[4]

These severe critiques of the disease model are more than enough to convince many that the model is a deeply problematic rhetorical frame for psychiatry.

What must be emphasized is that these critiques of the disease model are also critiques of the basic rhetorical frame of the *DSM-III*. They move beyond Kirk and Kutchins's bad-science critique and open up a science-as-usual critique of the *DSM-III*. In short, they challenge the basic rhetorical frame of the manual, and by doing so they challenge *DSM-III* developers' basic assumption that the disease model is the best rhetorical frame for psychiatry. With so many stakeholders so vehemently against the disease model, it cannot possibly be a good choice to make the disease model the *only* model of psychiatric diagnosis. But that is just what the *DSM-III* developers did. And with that choice, they made a serious mistake—so serious that it is fair to conclude only one thing: the *DSM-III* is not only bad science but also bad rhetoric. Very bad.

Bad Politics

It is not enough, however, to stay at either a "scientific" or a "rhetorical" level alone. Both of these levels remain too textual. They remain too caught up in books and articles, and they leave out the people involved in writing those texts. My reading of the *DSM-III* thus far reveals the tremendous contingency of the manual. Better science and better rhetoric, or at the very least different science and different rhetoric, would have taken the manual in dramatically different directions. To understand why the *DSM-III* emerged as the dominant text that it is, we must also examine the politics of the manual. We must go beyond textual analysis to what Foucault called "enunciative modalities" (see chap. 3). We have to animate the particular people of the *DSM-III*'s discourse and give them life.

Bruno Latour's work in science studies provides a valuable conceptual resource. In his discussion of ethnographies of science, Latour concludes that the "first rule of method" in studying seemingly neutral claims within science is to

> start with a textbook sentence which is devoid of any trace of fabrication, construction or ownership; we then put it in quotation marks, surround it with a bubble, place it in the mouth of someone who speaks; then we place them all in a specific situation, somewhere in time and space, surrounded by equipment, machines, colleagues; then when the controversy heats up a bit we look to where the disputing people go and what sort of new element they fetch, recruit or seduce in order to convince their colleagues; then we see how the people being convinced stop discussing with one another; situations, localizations, even people start being slowly erased; on the last picture we see a new sentence, without any quotation marks, written in a textbook similar to the one we started with in the first picture. (1987, 15)

Latour's first rule of method takes "neutral" scientific discourse out of its textual form and puts it in a cartoon-style bubble over the mouth of the speaker. In this way, Latour puts scientific claims back into the "mouth of someone who speaks." From there, he follows what happens next—who listens, who recruits whom, who defects, who is seduced. Latour's first rule of method works to reanimate neutral scientific discourse and helps open the door for a move from a scientific or rhetorical analysis to a *political analysis* of individuals and groups.

A political analysis of science is an extension of the science-as-usual critique. Typical scientific method only allows bad-science critiques, because it assumes it will be sufficient if the participants follow the methods of science. Going beyond bad-science critiques to science-as-usual critiques, we can also question basic rhetorical assumptions of science (as we did earlier), and we can question the political relations of the participants. A science-as-usual critique that focuses on political issues directs our attention to who gets included in the process. Who gets to sit at the table? Who gets to contribute? Who is excluded? What perspectives do they bring? And what effort is made to include alternative and additional perspectives?

Applying Latour's first rule to the *DSM-III*, we can begin a political critique of *DSM-III* by exploring who gets the new manual's bubble mouth and whom that mouth fetches, recruits, or seduces. Once again, Kirk and Kutchins provide valuable data. Though they do not pursue political issues directly (because they remain primarily focused on a scientific critique of the manual), Kirk and Kutchins do give ample information on the people involved in the manual. If we take their research and add the reports of published insider narratives, we get enough information to answer the "bubble-mouth" question for *DSM*.

Based on Kirk and Kutchins's research, the top *DSM-III* bubble mouth goes to Robert Spitzer. A career psychiatric researcher devoted to problems of nosology and classification, Spitzer was the leader of a group of Columbia University research psychiatrists. These psychiatrists were known for pioneering and developing structured interviews and objective diagnostic criteria. Allen Frances, the psychiatrist in charge of *DSM-IV*, described Spitzer as a "man whose entire life, private and public, personal and professional, is occupied with diagnosis and particularly with *DSM*" (Kirk and Kutchins 1992, 91).

Spitzer's involvement with the diagnostic manual came early in his career and dates back to the 1960s, when he was a major participant in developing *DSM-II*. After *DSM-II* was published, and despite his initial support and involvement, Spitzer became one of the manual's biggest antagonists. Spitzer published a 1974 paper offering a scathing critique of the diagnostic reliability of the *DSM-II*. Later that same year, he was chosen to head the *DSM-III* task force. Kirk and Kutchins argue that Spitzer's task-force appointment was "one of the most important committee assignments in psychiatry in the twentieth century" and that his "role cannot be ignored in any discussion of the evolution of modern psychiatric diagnosis" (1992, 63, 90).

Spitzer wrote the introduction for *DSM-III*, and it is from this text that I have chosen the quote to be "bubblized":

DSM-III reflects an increased commitment in our field to reliance on data as the basis for understanding mental disorders. . . . [Because of this], a series of field trials were conducted, beginning in 1977 and culminating in a two-year NIMH-sponsored field trial from September 1977 to September 1979. In all 12,667 patients were evaluated by approximately 550 clinicians, 474 of whom were in 212 different facilities, using successive drafts of *DSM-III.* . . . The results indicated that the great majority of participants, regardless of theoretical orientation, had a favorable response to *DSM-III.* (American Psychiatric Association 1980, 1, 5).

This is the official narrative of *DSM-III*'s development. If we put a bubble around the quote and clearly identify it with the voice and perspective of Robert Spitzer, we can begin to give the manual a more politically thick background.

Within four months of Spitzer's selection as chair of the *DSM-III* task force, he had fetched (recruited or seduced) all the members of the new committee. The members he chose consisted of a group of five psychiatrists. All had similar research interests, and all believed that psychiatric diagnosis should be based on allegedly theory-neutral objective criteria. One of the members, George Saslow, was known in psychiatry for his coauthored 1965 work entitled "Behavioral Diagnosis" (Kanfer and Saslow 1965). Two other members, Spitzer himself and one of his colleagues, Donald Klein, were known for promoting bioscience psychiatry and objective approaches to diagnosis. The two remaining members, Nancy Andreasen (who is now the editor of the leading professional journal in psychiatry and coauthor of the major psychiatric textbook I discuss in chap. 3) and Robert Woodruff, were associated with a team of psychiatric researchers at Washington University in St. Louis. Like Spitzer's Columbia group, the St. Louis researchers were devoted to operational psychiatric nosology and precise objective criteria for diagnosis. This kind of highly scientistic approach to psychiatry represented a narrow section of psychiatry. The committee members were, in Kirk and Kutchins's terms, a "minority among a minority" (1992, 49, 98).

Thus, Spitzer's task force was composed of an "invisible college" of like-minded researchers chosen from a narrow band of available possibilities (Kirk and Kutchins 1992, 98). They represented a new direction for psychiatry, and they were so aggressively sure of the superiority of their methods that they referred to themselves as the "Young Turks."

These young turks made it their project not only to redo the manual but to revamp psychiatry (Kirk and Kutchins 1992, 81). In 1978, psychiatrist Gerald Klerman dubbed these psychiatrists "Neo-Kraepelinians" and outlined the young turks' implicit "credo." Klerman's outline of the neo-Kraepelinian credo is worth quoting in full because it demonstrates the overlap between the diagnostic mind-set of the *DSM-III* task force and the disease model I describe earlier. According to Klerman, the neo-Kraepelinian credo includes the following beliefs:

1 Psychiatry is a branch of medicine.
2. Psychiatry should utilize modern scientific methodologies and base its practice on scientific knowledge.
3. Psychiatry treats people who are sick and who require treatment for mental illness.
4. There is a boundary between normal and sick.
5. There are discrete mental illnesses. Mental illnesses are not myths. There is not one but many mental illnesses. It is the task of scientific psychiatry, as of other medical specialties, to investigate the causes, diagnosis, and treatment of these mental illnesses.
6. The focus of psychiatric physicians should be particularly on the biological aspects of mental illnesses.
7. There should be an explicit and intentional concern with diagnosis and classification.
8. Diagnostic criteria should be codified, and a legitimate and valued area of research should be to validate such criteria by various techniques. Further, departments of psychiatry in medical schools should teach these criteria and not depreciate them, as has been the case for many years.
9. In research efforts directed at improving the reliability and validity of diagnosis and classification, statistical techniques should be utilized. (Qtd. in Kirk and Kutchins 1992, 50)

As this credo demonstrates, the stakes for psychiatry were high. Spitzer's *DSM-III* task force was not simply developing a new scientific nosology; it was also creating a new kind of psychiatry. Cleansed of subtlety, conflict, ambivalence, and uncertainty, neo-Kraepelinian scientific psychiatry is a polemic that passes itself off as neutral, and the eventual success of this disease model for psychiatry was wrapped up in the eventual success of *DSM-III*.

Spitzer's choice of membership for the initial task force demonstrates an added dimension of neo-Kraepelinian theoretical cleansing. Spitzer was not only cleansing ideas; he was cleansing people. Spitzer's cleansing was not so much ethnic cleansing (at least not on a manifest level) as perspectival cleansing. Spitzer's task force carefully eliminated any people with alternative perspectives—including the psychoanalytical psychotherapy perspective, which dominated psychiatry at that time—to create a mono-perspective committee. Kirk and Kutchins put it this way: "Among the five original psychiatrists on the task force, there was a remarkable congruence of interest. More importantly, there were no major divergent viewpoints, and the primary psychodynamic perspectives in psychiatry had no representative at the table" (1992, 98).

Once Spitzer recruited his task force, he wasted no time reworking the manual in his neo-Kraepelinian image. Within one year after the *DSM-III* task force was formed, they completed the first draft of the new manual. The draft was officially tentative, but it was no mere rough draft or provisional starting point. It successfully incorporated all the major innovations that were eventually included in *DSM-III*. As Kirk and Kutchins point out, "Although another five years passed before the manual was published, the essential decisions about its approach, structure, and contents were made quickly by Spitzer and this small group" (1992, 99). All the basic conceptual schemata and distinctive features of the new manual were put in place by this powerful and strategically placed minority of like-minded psychiatrists.

After such a quick start, what happened over the next five years? To put it bluntly, during this period the task force covered its tracks. The initial draft was followed by a long, tortuous process of refining the manual and obtaining official approval. Key to this process was the use of field trials to test the manual. I have already discussed Kirk and Kutchins's concern regarding the exaggerated scientific claims of the field trials. Here, I want to highlight how the field-trial approach to verification focused on testing already created categories rather than the actual creation of categories. This emphasis on testing effectively covered over the fact that only a very narrow band of participants were involved in the manual's initial creation.

Spitzer says that "12,667 patients were evaluated by approximately 550 clinicians," and the back appendix of the *DSM-III* lists hundreds of contributors to the manual. This gives the appearance of a broad base of involvement and participation in the manual's production. However, almost all of these names (all but five) are of people who were involved in the field trials rather than of people involved in the initial draft of the manual. These people "tested" the manual according to the rules, norms, and priorities of the initial task force. They did not participate in the creation of the manual. Thus, the five-year period between the *DSM-III*'s initial draft and its subsequent ratification and publication gives the false impression that the manual was developed by a broad base within the psychiatric stakeholder community. The truth was just the opposite. The manual represented the forced will of a very few people and an extremely limited number of psychiatric stakeholders.

And it was not only psychodynamic perspectives that got shut out. So did psychology perspectives, social work perspectives, and other mental health perspectives (Schacht 1985). In addition to professional exclusions like these, *DSM-III* developers also excluded pretty much anyone who was not a privileged, white, male, academic psychiatrist (Malik and Beutler 2002, 6). The most detailed account of these exclusionary practices comes from insider exposés written by feminist psychologist Paula Caplan. In her book *They Say You're Crazy: How the World's Most Powerful Psychiatrists Decide Who's Normal*, Caplan gives a detailed account of the relational dynamics of the manual (1995). She describes the responses she and a group of feminist researchers (therapists, psychologists, and psychiatrists) received when they attempted to contribute to the manual. Throughout the process, they were systematically snubbed, ignored, denigrated, and dismissed.

Caplan and her colleagues got involved with the manual after becoming concerned that key diagnoses under consideration, such as one describing "masochism" (or "self-defeating personality disorder") and one describing "premenstrual dysphoria," were riddled with sexist assumptions. Like Kirk and Kutchins, Caplan couched her concerns in the form of a bad-science critique. She reviewed the scientific literature for these proposed diagnoses and found herself in deep disagreement with the developers' perspective. She argued that these diagnoses were not diseases at all, but simply a pathologizing of culturally produced gender patterns. When she tried to get her scientific conclusions to the *DSM* developers, she was politely but persistently rebuffed and excluded.

Caplan and her colleagues went beyond critiques of the manual's premenstrual and self-defeating personality diagnoses. They also proposed some diagnoses of their own. For Caplan and her colleagues, if the diagnostic manual was going to pathologize culturally produced femininity, then it should be consistent and do the same for masculinity. But when

Caplan and her colleagues suggested some parallel diagnoses, like "testosterone induced aggression" and "macho personality disorder" (which they called "delusional dominating personality disorder"), they got even less respect and were refused even the semblance of an audience.

According to Caplan's own report, she worked hard to think the best of the *DSM* developers. She was very reluctant to see them as a narrow-minded interest group, and she thought if they could just see good arguments and good data they would come around. Eventually, however, she had to give up her sense that the developers were just doing neutral science. Clearly, they had an agenda, and feminist concerns were not part of it. Rather than argue the merits of the competing claims, the developers stonewalled and excluded their opponents. Caplan categorized the various stonewalling and exclusionary procedures used by the *DSM* developers, and she came up with twenty-five different gate-keeping methods. These ranged from nonresponsiveness, to bait-and-switch tactics, to outright lying and manipulation (Caplan 1995, 222). The stonewalling tactics not only kept out feminist concerns but were also used to fight resistance to other highly problematic diagnoses, like "ego-dystonic homosexuality," and to avoid any serious consideration of a "racist personality disorder" diagnosis (Caplan 1995, 221).

I should note that there was some shift in the developers' exclusionary practices from *DSM-III* to *DSM-IV*. After receiving much criticism on the issue, *DSM-IV* developers were much more sensitive to charges that the *DSM-III* was exclusionary. As a result, they promoted an increased air of "inclusiveness" from the *DSM-III* to the *DSM-IV* (Nathan 1998). But these changes seem to be more window dressing than real inclusiveness. The *DSM-IV* developers' efforts to include women and racial and ethnic minorities, as well as nonpsychiatric mental health professionals, made little difference in the overall perspective of the next edition of the manual. Since there was no serious rethinking of the manual from the *DSM-III* to the *DSM-IV*, there would be little room for alternative perspectives to actually get in to the manual. And if that were not enough, the inclusion that did happen seemed to be more about including diverse body types rather than genuinely diverse perspectives. Indeed, most of the difficulties that Caplan describes in getting a feminist perspective into the manual involve struggles she had with *DSM-IV* developers—many of whom, at least in the subcommittees that Caplan was working with, were women. Just because more "women" are let into science, that does not mean that more feminists are let into science. *DSM-IV* is no exception.

Caplan and Kirk and Kutchins give us enough information to sketch out the politics of *DSM-III*'s development, but their motivation for doing so is largely wrapped up in a bad-science critique. For both Caplan and Kirk and Kutchins, the relevance of these internal psychiatric politics is that they created bad science and distorted data. But bad science and distorted data are not the whole problem. The *autocratic and exclusionary politics* used by the *DSM* developers must be critiqued directly. Otherwise, the situation perpetually repeats itself. By staying within a "bad-science" critique, Caplan and Kirk and Kutchins make it seem as if there would be no problem if the developers had only agreed with them. But that misses a major issue. These autocratic and exclusionary political tactics are at the core of *DSM-III* and *DSM-IV*. They go straight back to the initial political style set by Robert Spitzer. Changes in the details of the manual will not change this issue. The politics of *DSM* must be changed directly. Spitzer's autocratic style is a problem not only because it led to bad science but more fundamentally because his politics are bad in themselves. In other words, Spitzer's politics are bad (have bad consequences) for psychiatry because his politics are bad—too authoritarian and too antidemocratic.

At this level of political critique, the science question and even the rhetorical question are only part of the problem. They are surface manifestations of deeper political problems. Spitzer and the neo-Kraepelinians must also be critiqued on political grounds. Kirk and Kutchins have shown us that Spitzer's science was bad, and my review of alternative rhetorical options shows that their rhetoric was bad. But improving future *DSM* developers' science and rhetoric will not improve their politics. That will require specific and direct attention to the politics of science and knowledge in psychiatry.

Just a quick peak into the planned *DSM-V* will give a sense of what I mean. Preliminary *DSM-V* research planning activities can be found in David Kupfer, Michael First, and Darrel Regier's book *A Research Agenda for DSM-V* (2002), and ongoing information can be found at the *DSM-V* Prelude Project Web site (http://www.dsm5.org/index.cfm). One of the most striking things about these early efforts toward creating the *DSM-V* is how willing the developers are to open up questions of science and even rhetoric, at least up to a point. Please do not get me wrong: the developers remain within a very narrow scientistic frame. The goal of the *DSM-V,* as the new developers put it, is to "enrich [the] empirical data base" and to incorporate scientific research findings from "animal studies, genetics, neuroscience, epidemiology, clinical research, cross-cultural research, and clinical services research" (see http://dsm5.org/whitepapers.cfm). But within that scientistic frame, the developers say clearly that an "improved scientific basis" for the *DSM* will likely require major changes. Indeed, they expect it to require "as yet unknown paradigm shifts" (Kupfer, First, and Regier 2002, xix).

Although the new "paradigm" remains uncertain, all indications suggest that the developers plan to move the *DSM-V* from a syndrome-based perspective to a pathophysiology-based one. The new developers set the stage for this by lamenting that current *DSM* categories are "devoid of biology." As such, they plan to develop a system that incorporates multiple forms of biological markers. These markers, they argue, will allow psychiatry to finally achieve more than "reliability." Through a pathophysiological system, psychiatry can achieve "valid" psychiatric diagnoses that do not shy away from etiological explanations.

The domains in which the developers plan to look for etiological diagnostic categories include: "1) better animal models for the major psychiatric disorders; 2) genes that help determine abnormal behavior in animal models; 3) imaging studies in animals to better understand the nature of imaged signals in humans; and 4) functional genomics and proteomics involved in psychiatric disorders, that is the identification of genes or proteins that are regulated in particular brain regions by a given drug or behavioral state." In addition, they plan to include: "1) work to identify disease-related genes from among the 26,000 identified in the human genome project; 2) post-mortem studies to examine circuitry and gene expression; 3) the newer brain imaging techniques; 4) approaches that integrate the use of multiple modalities; and 5) neuroinfomatics, the integration and management of large amounts of data produced at various levels of investigation" (see http://dsm5.org/whitepapers.cfm).

The genius of this plan is that, should the developers succeed, they will dramatically throw up for revision both the basic science and the rhetorical frame (or paradigmatic model) of the *DSM*, while still staying within the same larger scientist episteme. But for all their openness to change and exploration, what the developers are not throwing up for consideration is the question of politics. Who gets to sit at the table of the creation of *DSM-V*? Why are these people chosen? What kinds of efforts are made to generate diversity? Who gets selected to leadership positions? What kinds of authority do they have? How are differences approached? There is no sign that these questions are given any systematic thought. All the systematic thought goes into questions of content. None goes into the question of process and inclusion.

Interestingly, there are some nonsystematic efforts at considering questions of inclusion. For example, the early planning conferences are being cochaired by a "distinguished investigator in the same field from a country other than the U.S." (see http://dsm5.org/planning.cfm). And there is some reaching into additional disciplines. For example, the developers tell us work-group members were selected "primarily for their expertise in diverse areas such as family and twin studies, molecular genetics, basic and clinical neuroscience, cognitive and behavioral science, development, life span issues, disability, psychopathology, and treatment. In order to encourage thinking beyond the current DSM-IV framework, most of the workgroup members had not been closely involved in the DSM-IV development process" (see http://dsm5.org/whitepapers.cfm). But by what criteria were these efforts at diversity made? Why these new members and not others?

These kinds of inclusion gestures do not come close to a systematic consideration of difference and inclusion. They seem much more like strategically manipulative inclusions based on very narrow special interests. Do the developers really believe that adding different *DSM* developers from these "diverse areas" will truly "encourage thinking beyond the current DSM-IV framework"? It seems that they do, but only along very constricted lines.

As a result, the emergent *DSM-V* will in all likelihood both dramatically change and fundamentally stay the same. It will change in its content, but it will stay the same in its basic scientistic frame and its fundamental power relations. *DSM-V* will rearrange the science and rhetoric but not change the critical problems with a narrowly scientistic disease-model approach. Nor will it change in any meaningful way its elitist and autocratic politics of inclusion.

Conclusion

Kirk and Kutchins provide invaluable tools for critiquing psychiatry's new diagnostic manual. Their work effectively critiques the fundamental scientific premise—increased reliability—on which that manual stands. However, although Kirk and Kutchins's critique is wide-ranging, and although it purports to address the "rhetoric of science," it falls short on both the rhetorical and the political dimensions of the new manual. In

Sandra Harding's terminology, Kirk and Kutchins do a bad-science critique that leaves *DSM-III* science-as-usual unquestioned. Kirk and Kutchins do not seriously challenge the basic assumptions of the manual. They do not challenge the basic rhetorical frame of the manual or the political practices of its developers. From a postpsychiatry perspective, these additional rhetorical and political critiques are exactly what must happen, and science-as-usual in psychiatry must change.

This reading of *DSM* shows that contemporary science-as-usual is creating an exclusionary approach to psychiatric diagnostic research that does not include or respect alternative perspectives. In the next chapter, I move from the *DSM* to Prozac. If we now have some idea what's been going on with the *DSM*, the next cultural studies of psychiatry question I ask is this: *What in the world happened with the advent of Prozac?*

CHAPTER SEVEN

Prozac & the Posthuman
Politics of Cyborgs

I phoned my editor and left a message on her voice mail. I said, I
know you are tired of hearing this sort of thing from authors, but
something *unusual* is happening out here.
—Peter Kramer, *Listening to Prozac* (italics added)

The Epidemic of Prozac Signification

The first edition of Peter Kramer's *Listening to Prozac* came out in 1993.
As it happened, it made it to the bookstores about the same time as that
year's American Psychiatric Convention. Kramer, a psychiatrist and new
book author, was so excited about being in print that he ran to a book-
store near the convention to see himself in print. He found the book selling out as soon as a new shipment arrived: "The staff had unpacked some
copies that morning, but they were sold out. . . . When I returned the
reshipments had come and gone. I never did manage to catch the books:
as soon as they arrived, they were snatched up" (Kramer 1997, 315). *Listening to Prozac* turned out to be a national best seller, but at the time
Kramer was surprised and elated by the success of his book. He franti-
cally called his editor to tell her that something *unusual* was going on.

With the advantage of hindsight, we now know that Kramer was right:
something unusual was going on with Prozac. But what, exactly, was that
something unusual? At the time, the Prozac craze of the 1990s was just
getting started, and the fever pitch of the moment made it difficult to

interpret Prozac. But now that the hype has passed, Prozac has come off patent, and the pressured commentary has dissipated, it is easier to get a perspective on the something unusual of Prozac. Indeed, it is now possible to begin a serious cultural study of Prozac.

Clearly part of the something unusual of Prozac was the incredible epidemic of Prozac prescribing. The Food and Drug Administration first gave Eli Lilly the marketing go-ahead for Prozac in 1987. By 1993, new U.S. prescriptions had climbed to 7.6 million. By 2002, the year after Prozac came off patent, that number reached over 27 million. If you combine Prozac prescriptions with those of the multiple "me-too" drugs it inspired—the class of antidepressants known as "selective serotonin inhibitors" (SSRIs)—the total reaches 67.5 million new prescriptions in the United States alone (Alliance for Human Protection, 2004). This means that almost one in four people in the United States were started on a Prozac-type SSRI between 1988 and 2002. No matter how you look at it, a major part of the Prozac story was its status as a blockbuster drug spawning an incredible epidemic of antidepressant prescriptions.

But the number of prescriptions was only part of the "something unusual" of Prozac. Beyond the epidemic of prescriptions, another key part of the Prozac story was the simultaneous *epidemic of signification* that grew up around the medication.[1] Representations of Prozac exploded during those years. In medical and psychiatric literature alone, there were 4,654 Medline citations of Prozac between 1987 and 2002. Prozac was also a frequent topic in the mass media and the popular press (Montagne 2001, 2002). The drug was on the cover of *Newsweek, Time,* and the *New Yorker,* and it was often featured on the talk-show circuit of Oprah, Geraldo, and Phil. In addition to Kramer's *Listening to Prozac,* Prozac was the star of a host of other popular texts: *Talking Back to Prozac* (Breggin 1994), *Prozac Nation* (Wurtzel 1994), *Prozac Diary* (Slater 1998), *Prozac Highway* (Blackbridge 1999), and *Beyond Prozac* (1996), to name a few. And if that were not enough, Prozac even spawned its own video game called Virtual Prozac. In short, Prozac commentary and Prozac representation were everywhere during the 1990s.

Out of the cacophony of voices, commentators from many different backgrounds tried to sum up the "something unusual" of Prozac. Consider the following examples. From the *Handbook of Psychiatric Drug Therapy:*

> The recognition that specific neuronal uptake mechanisms for serotonin were present in the CNS [Central Nervous System] suggested, as early as the late 1960s, a potential target for the development of antidepressants. By the early 1970s, the technology existed for the

screening of molecules that could selectively inhibit serotonin uptake. In 1972, fluozetine (Prozac) was shown to produce selective inhibition of serotonin uptake in rat synaptosomes. This drug, the first in its class . . . was approved for release in the United States in December 1987. [Its] impact . . . on the treatment of depression has been extraordinary, with more than 10 million people prescribed . . . by 1994. The success appears to derive mainly from side effect advantages over older agents . . . [and has] generated wide patient and prescriber acceptance. (Hyman, Arana, and Rosenbaum 1995, 62)

From *Psychology Today:*

Slowly, stealthily, Prozac is slithering into more and more of our lives and finding a warm place to settle. Even the most casually aware citizen can feel the shift in thinking brought about by the drug's ability to "transform" its users: We speak of personality change; we argue over the drug's benefits over psychotherapy (all those expensive hours of parent-bashing as compared to a monthly dash to the pharmacy); and we let ourselves imagine a world in which our pain is nullified, erased as easily and fully as dirty words on a school blackboard. (Mauro 1994, 44)

From the *Tribune Business News:*

Feeling despondent? Beset by burning stomachaches? Are your arteries hopelessly clogged? Well, you're not alone. Prescription medications for depression, ulcers, and high cholesterol dominated the list of best-selling drugs last year with six of the top ten entries. . . . What's more, these half-dozen drugs generated $8.1 billion, or an impressive 9.5% of the $85.4 billion in prescription drugs sold in 1996. . . . Overall, the sale of prescription drugs to pharmacies rose by 10% in 1996. . . . Eli Lilly's Prozac was the third leading bestseller overall with sales of 1.7 billion, a 14% rise [from 1995]. . . . Pfizer's Zoloft was fifth with sales of $ 1.1 billion. (Silverman 1997, 216)

From Andrew Weil's *New York Times* best seller *Spontaneous Healing:*

What about depression, which is now epidemic in our culture? I experience depression as a state of higher potential energy, wound up and turned inward on itself. If that energy can be accessed and moved, it can be a catalyst for spontaneous healing. The psychiatric profession treats depression almost exclusively by prescribing drugs, especially a new class of antidepressants called serotonin reuptake inhibitors, of which Prozac is a prototype. The pharmaceutical industry markets these drugs aggressively and successfully, partly by convincing people that they cannot know their full human potential unless they use them. Recently a woman friend of mine in her early fifties went for a routine checkup to her gynecologist, also a woman. After the examination was over, the gynecologist asked her, "Well, do you want me to write you a prescription for Prozac?" "Why should I want to take Prozac?" my friend replied. "I'm not depressed." "How do you know?" asked the doctor. (1995, 201)

With this kind of interpretive diversity, the basic cultural studies question is this: How can, or should, we interpret the Prozac story in light of this epidemic of signification? Is the *Handbook of Psychiatric Drug Therapy* right about the something unusual of Prozac? Is Prozac a straightforward example of medical progress? Or is *Psychology Today* more on target? Is Prozac a complex cultural phenomenon? Or perhaps the *Tribune Business News* has the best interpretation. Perhaps Prozac is just good business. But then again, Andrew Weil seems to be onto something important as well. Perhaps Prozac is best seen as symptomatic of a medical system out of touch with healing and obsessed with technology and profits. How, in other words, should the Prozac story be narrated with such a diversity of options? Is Prozac progress or regress—panacea or Pandora? Should the clinical-science literature have the final say on this question? If not, why not? What are the cultural issues of Prozac signification? What are the political ones? Who should answer these questions, for whom, and with what claim to legitimacy?

The Time of Cyborgs

To approach these questions and to get some additional perspective on the Prozac phenomenon, let me start by considering the Prozac story within the context of a range of new science and technology—or techno-science for short—that has dramatically infiltrated many of our daily lives. Just think about the amount of time you spend in some kind of synergistic interface with a machine. How much time in your day are you *not* on the telephone, at the computer, watching TV, listening to the radio, in the car, on the train, or in a climate-controlled environment? How many thousands of advertisements and commercials have you seen in which happiness is promised through a technological interface—a long-distance phone call, an exciting new car, an opportunity to sit by the ocean (simultaneously connected to a global network on your personal laptop computer)? These messages are always the same—technology enhances life and brings smiles . . . *for a price.*

Increasingly, technoscience has infiltrated medicine too. Although technology in medicine is not new, the recent explosion of technical capacities in medicine has created a qualitative shift in the practice of medicine (Rifkin 1998; Parens 1998; Fukuyama 2002; Elliot 2003; President's Council on Bioethics 2003). Indeed, we may increasingly understand medicine as a kind of applied technoscience. New biotechnologies—including advanced imaging techniques, genetic manipulations, organ transplantation, artificial limbs, expanding cosmetic surgeries, and an array of new psychopharmaceuticals—have rapidly turned medicine into technomedicine. Not only has technoscience become a staple of medical diagnosis and treatment, but technoscience has also catapulted medicine into an era of physical and mental enhancement. With the further developments of the dawning biotech century, everything from the human life span, to mental and physical abilities, to personality will be molded in ways that were previously unimaginable. In this environment, physicians and psychiatrists are in danger of becoming glorified distributors of the new technologies—sort of like new-car dealers with a medical certificate.

The recent epidemics of Prozac prescribing and Prozac signification are located in the center of this explosion of technomedicine. Indeed, Prozac was one of the first of the new psychopharmaceuticals to sit uncomfortably between a treatment and an enhancement, between a medication and a mental cosmetic. In Kramer's words, Prozac ushered in the dawn of "cosmetic psychopharmachology" (1997, xvi; Giannini 2004). But, as helpful as it may be to locate Prozac within the new technomedicine, this contextualization does not solve all of our interpretive problems. Unfortunately, technomedicine is also not well understood. The technomedical invasion has happened so fast that the standard medical literature has not caught up with the full complexities of medicine as technoscience. Nor has it even begun to develop a critical discourse of this phenomenon.

Before further embracing the joys and smiles of technoscience body enhancement, medical and psychiatric scholars must seek a discursive enhancement to better understand and better cope with the rise of technomedicine. One discursive option I have found extremely useful in sorting through the Prozac story is the work of cultural studies of science scholar Donna Haraway. If asked, Haraway might categorize herself as a postmodern feminist science historian of the present. In her writings, she has initiated a great expansion of the cyborg metaphor, and she is a major initiator of what many are calling cyber-feminism and others are calling posthumanism (Braidotti 1994, 102; Halberstam and Livingston 1995; Kirkup et al. 2000). For Haraway's cyborg metaphor to make sense, however, it is helpful to explain what I mean by "metaphor" in this context. The surest way to misunderstand Haraway's work is to approach it too "literally" or too "metaphorically" without rethinking the usual meanings of these terms.

Haraway (in the company of most postmodern philosophers and antifoundational theorists, and consistent with my discussions of theory in the first four chapters) reverses, rejects, and ultimately displaces the notion that "metaphorical" meaning can be understood as distinct from "literal" meaning. According to Haraway, there are not "metaphorical" meanings and "literal" meanings (separable on deep ontological or epistemological grounds); there are only different possible meaning formations. For Haraway, the proper questions for particular meaning formations (like bioscience), which are always already metaphorical and literal, are not simply scientific and epistemological questions of whether the meanings mirror the world independent of human constructs. Rather, the proper questions are also ethical and political questions of what world this kind of meaning formation will create. What effects will this meaning formation have on particular living narratives, and who or what is benefiting (and why) by making meaning this way rather than another way?

Thus, when Haraway says, "By the late twentieth century, our time, a mythic time, we are all chimeras, theorized and fabricated hybrids of machine and organism; in short we are cyborgs. The cyborg is our ontology; it gives us our politics" (1991, 150), she means to be both literal and metaphorical at the same time. For Haraway, there is a literal truth to her cyborg claim—something worth struggling and fighting over—and simultaneously the cyborg metaphor is an "imaginative resource suggesting some very fruitful couplings" (1991, 150). In other words, cyborgs make for productive thinking in the current age of dramatic technoscience proliferation. But what are cyborgs? For Haraway, cyborgs are cybernetic organisms—systems that embrace living and technological components. Since the cyborg is always and inseparably organic and machinic, the cyborg displaces, and renders nonessential, crusty West-

ern binaries like nature/culture, fact/value, pure/contaminated, inor-
ganic/organic, and real/artificial. These distinctions, while useful in the
past, do not work well in the current technoscience moment—which
effectively blurs them all.

Haraway uses the cyborg to enter the fray of science politics not by
arguing for a repudiation of science or technology (it is way too late for
that) but by arguing for mixing up the scientific and technological with
the cultural, political, and aesthetic. Considering herself a "child of
antiracist, feminist, multicultural, and radical science movements," Haraway "yearns for knowledge, freedom, and justice *within* the world of science and technology" (1997, 267, italics added). For Haraway, cyborgs
effectively cut through much of the theoretical baggage associated with
technoscience binary thinking that can inhibit her yearning. The issue
for Haraway is not *whether* the organic and machinic are mixed, but *how*
they are mixed and to what effect. Who is doing the mixing, and who is
being affected? What are the social and political relations between the
participants and the stakeholders? For Haraway, we may all be cyborgs,
but not all cyborg mixings are the same.

Haraway argues that behind the seemingly "natural" evidence of a sup-
posedly objective scientific method, biomedical science is not only culturally constructed but also big politics and big business. "Biology," she
reminds us, "is not the body itself but a discourse of the body" (1997,
217). For Haraway, bioscience discourse is far from neutral (and far
from "progressive") in its political and cultural alliances in what she calls
the "New World Order, Inc." (1997, 2). Indeed, bioscience, while legiti-
mating itself with a rhetoric of "new scientific progress," is simultaneously bedfellows with many of the old politically regressive power structures of patriarchy, racism, classism, ableism, neocolonialism, and
homophobia. These alliances remain invisible, however, if bioscience is
able to proceed free and aloof from other critical discourse; free from
deep and serious cultural and political questioning, not only about the
technical applications of bioscience but also about what projects to take
up, who should develop them, and what consequences follow from
handing over so much authority to a realm of scientific world-making
independent of democratic politics.

The Cultural Dynamics of Prozac

With Haraway's cultural studies of science in mind, let me return to the
Prozac story. What is the relevance of the cyborg metaphor for the
recent epidemic of Prozac prescribing and Prozac signification? How do

we go from theoretical analysis to practical cultural analysis? How can we interpret the cultural meaning and legitimacy of Prozac (and other psychopharmaceuticals dominant in psychiatry—which Prozac metonymically represents)? Who are the "we" who will do all of this?

For starters, Haraway's cyborg theory helps us sort out *what will not work*. From a cyborg perspective, neither of the standard discourses of science or bioethics can fully interpret the Prozac story. Prozac, like all technoscience, turns out to be too slippery, too contradictory, too coyote wily, for the broad-brush discourses of science and ethics to fully understand. Neither science nor ethics alone can come close to sorting through the Prozac phenomenon.

Scientific discourse, in particular, has had great difficulty reaching interpretive conclusions about Prozac. In the thirty years since the Prozac compound—Lilly 110140 3-(p-trifluoromethylphenoxy)-N-methyl-3-phenylpropylamine—was first studied, scientific research has not been able to agree on even simple questions like: Does the drug work? Or, is it safe? The fact of this inability is true now, and it was true during the height of the Prozac-prescribing craze. In the middle 1990s, the third edition of the *Handbook of Psychiatric Drug Therapy* (Hyman, Arana, and Rosenbaum 1995) claimed with great certainty and authority that Prozac was highly effective. Typical of most clinical-science reviews, the handbook concluded that "[Prozac] is clearly effective for major depression" (1995, 64). In a glowing review, the authors estimated that "for those who meet DSM-IV criteria for major depression, it can be expected that approximately 50% will fully recover. . . . Of the remainder, the majority will show some degree of improvement" (1995, 47). Also typical of most clinical-science reviews, the handbook minimized the drug's side effects. It mentioned anxiety, agitation, nausea, headaches, sexual dysfunction, and occasionally apathy (1995, 65) but downplayed these, concluding that the overall side-effect profile was highly favorable for the drugs: "the absence of anticholinergic, antihstiaminergic, anti-alpha-adrenergic, weight gain, and cardio-toxic effects and potential for lethality in overdose [results in] wide patient and prescriber acceptance" (1995, 62).

In direct opposition to such clinical-science conclusions, other scientific analyses concluded that Prozac (1) was minimally effective *and* (2) had very serious side effects. Regarding efficacy, many scientists reviewing the data found that Prozac was not much better than a sugar pill in treating depression (see, e.g., Breggin 1994, 65; Fisher and Fisher 1996). In 1998, psychologists Irving Kirsch and Guy Sapirstein did an extensive meta-analysis of the efficacy literature. They looked at nineteen double-blind studies involving over two thousand patients. Kirsch and Sapirstein concluded that inactive placebos produced 75 percent of Prozac's efficacy. And not only that, but they also speculated that the other 25 percent came largely from nonspecific side effects. As Kirsch and Sapirstein put it, most researchers were "listening to Prozac but hearing placebo" (1998).

This efficacy controversy continues to this day. Some champion SSRIs; some believe they hardly work at all. So far, there are no signs of resolution on the horizon. After Kirsch and Sapirstein published their meta-analysis, their conclusions were disputed in the medical literature by D. Klein and F. Quitkin (Klein 1998; Quitkin et al. 2000). Kirsch, joined by several other colleagues, responded to Klein and Quitkin with a follow-up study that reasserted the earlier findings (Kirsch et al. 2002). The popular press also picked up the placebo controversy and ran a series of stories with titles like "Maybe It's All in Your Head," "Make-Believe Medicine," "Antidepressants: Hype or Help," and "Misguided Medicine: A Stunning Finding about Antidepressants Is Being Ignored." The most extensive of these popular-press stories ran in the *Washington Post* and was entitled "Against Depression: A Sugar Pill Is Hard to Beat" (Vedantam 2002). *Post* reporter S. Vedantam emphasized the placebo side of the controversy, but researchers Brandon Gaudiano and James Herbert disputed Vedantam's main claims (2003). They warned that the recent media flurry risks overhyping the "power" of placebos and the "powerlessness" of antidepressants like Prozac.

Science has done no better in answering the side-effect question. If anything, the mainstream clinical-science assessment that Prozac has few side effects has been even more controversial than the efficacy question. Most of the side-effect controversy has centered on questions of sexual dysfunction and suicidality. As we saw above, the *Handbook of Psychiatric Drug Therapy* mentions sexual side effects but effectively downplays these problems. Eli Lilly, in its product information, claims that sexual dysfunctions occurred in only 2–5 percent of patients. Lilly based this number on its clinical trials of the medication. But when psychiatrist Joseph Glenmullen reviewed the scientific literature, he concluded that sexual dysfunction occurred in 60 percent of patients (2000, 107).

As for the side effects of suicide, and even violence, these risks were not mentioned in the handbook or the product information. But outside mainstream clinical literature, this side effect haunted Prozac all through the 1990s. This serious potential of suicide and violence was first raised most clearly by psychiatrist Peter Breggin (1994). It was further corroborated by psychiatric researcher David Healy (1997, 2004). The mainstream literature denied or minimized these concerns throughout the 1990s, but now the tide of opinion has turned around completely. The possibility of serious side effects has become so widely credible that class-action lawsuits against the makers of Prozac-type drugs have begun. These suits seek damages against the pharmaceutical companies for withholding information on these serious side effects (Alliance for Health and Human Research 2004; "Editorial" 2004; "Analysis" 2004; Healy 2004; see also http://www.injuryboard.com).[2]

In addition, the issue of efficacy and safety has yet further complications. Even if the safety and efficacy questions were somehow resolved to everyone's agreement, and even if the resolution were in favor of Prozac-type drugs, that would not mean there is less need for cultural analysis of the medication. Just the opposite, it would mean that it was needed even more. As Francis Fukuyama puts it, "the more difficult political and moral problem will occur if Prozac is found to be completely safe and if it, or similar drugs yet discovered, work just as advertised" (2002, 44). In other words, when more effective and safe Prozac-type drugs hit the market (and there is no reason to believe this will not happen relatively soon), the spread of the medication will be even more dramatic.

Going beyond efficacy and safety, the other undecidable scientific question regarding Prozac-type drugs involves explanation. The question can be worded this way: for those who believe Prozac works, why does it work? Here again science has struggled miserably. It has been hopelessly lost trying to explain *why* the drug improves people's moods, if indeed it does. Some scientists argue vociferously that Prozac "works" because it treats a biological disease. To use the favored analogy of biopsychiatry, Prozac treats depression the way insulin treats diabetes. The diabetes analogy is supposed to work like this: the biological deficiency in diabetes is low insulin; similarly, the biological deficiency in depression is a neurotransmitter "chemical imbalance."

But others argue just as vociferously that the "chemical imbalance" analogy is all wet. For them, Prozac works (if it does work) simply because it is a psychic stimulant. They maintain that Prozac works on the same neurotransmitter systems that other stimulants (such as cocaine and amphetamines) work on, and thus they are similar mood brighteners and psychic energizers. Sigmund Freud described the stimulant effects of cocaine beautifully as far back as 1884. He found that cocaine produced

exhilaration and lasting euphoria, which in no way differs from the
normal euphoria of the healthy person. . . . You perceive an increase
of self-control and possess more vitality and capacity for work. . . . In
other words, you are simply normal, and it is hard to believe that you
are under the influence of any drug. . . . Long intensive mental or
physical work is performed without fatigue. . . . The result is enjoyed
without any of the unpleasant after effects that follow exhilaration
brought about by alcohol. (Qtd. in Breggin 1994, 116)

Over one hundred years later, former cocaine abusers report that Prozac
gives them the same feeling as a mild dose of cocaine: "So long as I
didn't do too much coke, if I just did a few lines, I would feel in a good
mood. It was only when I did too much or if I smoked it or shot it up
instead of snorting lines that I would feel really racy and strung out.
Prozac is like the milder effect, like just a line or two" (Glenmullen 2000,
213). If we understand Prozac as working like a mild stimulant, there is
no need to hypothesize about it treating a "mental disease" or a "chemical imbalance." Prozac just produces the stimulant effect of speed. It
would do so on anyone.

Like the discourse of science and the "true" of Prozac, the discourse of
bioethics has had little luck deciding if Prozac is "good." Ethicists generally parse the "good" from the "bad" in the case of a drug like Prozac
through a discursive logic that rides on a sharp distinction between
"therapy" and "enhancement." As the Presidents Council on Bioethics
puts it, therapy "is the use of biotechnical power to treat individuals with
known diseases, disabilities, or impairments, in an attempt to restore
them to a normal state of health and fitness" (2003, 13). By contrast,
enhancement is the "directed use of biotechnical power to alter, by
direct intervention, not disease processes but the 'normal' workings of
the human body and psyche, to augment or improve their native capacities and performances" (2003, 13) Using this distinction, if Prozac
involves medical treatment of an actual disease, then bioethicists would
generally consider it good (and believe that it should be supported and
funded). If it involves a mere cosmetic enhancement of the normal
workings of the brain, then they would consider it bad (and believe that
it should not be supported and funded). But of course, the scientific
controversy surrounding Prozac makes this distinction of little help.
Some scientists see Prozac as treating mental disease—the way insulin
treats diabetes—and some see it as enhancing moods and psychic
energy—like a mild dose of cocaine. This incommensurable, and there-

fore irresolvable, discursive dispute leaves it completely undecidable whether Prozac is a treatment or an enhancement.

Increasingly, ethicists attempt to avoid conundrums like this by moving "beyond the therapy/enhancement" binary (Parens 1998; Elliot 2003). Refreshingly, these ethicists enter the technomedical domain not by reproducing the treatment/enhancement distinction as a means to separate the "good" and the "bad" of medical technoscience. Carl Elliot, for example, considers instead the broad cultural and historical context of these new technologies. For Elliot, "we need to understand the complex relationship between enhancement technologies, the way we live now, and the kinds of people we have become" (2003, xxi). Elliot calls for an "ethics of authenticity," and he argues that the good and the bad of technologies like Prozac can be approached through deeper questions involving the meaning of life: "How should I live?" and "Am I being true to myself?" (1998, 182). His analysis extends not only to America's eager consumption of the new technologies but also to its lingering anxiety and unease about that consumption. He finds the American self replete with deep conflicts between the relentless pursuit of social status and insistent yearnings for authenticity. He finds Americans unable to negotiate these conflicts and highly vulnerable to the lure of medical enhancements. Such technologies promise improved social status at the same time they threaten feelings of authenticity.

Unfortunately, although this move effectively sidesteps the disease/enhancement binary, it gets stuck in a very similar dichotomy. Does Prozac create "real" or "honest" happiness? Does it make you "truly happy," as the President's Council on Bioethics puts it? Or does the drug create an inauthentic, artificial, shallow, and out-of-touch happiness? From Haraway's perspective, these kinds of efforts to create an "ethic of authenticity" have lost much of their purchase. Humanity (or what may be called "posthumanity" in a cyborg age) in the New World Order, Inc. is too intertwined with technoscience for these distinctions to be of much use. In the time of cyborgs, "real" or "honest" happiness outside of technoscience augmentation makes little practical sense. All happiness in the cyborg age is an irretrievable combination of real and artificial. As a result, the distinction no longer helps or provides meaningful guidance.

The difficulties that the discourses of science and ethics have in interpreting Prozac mean that these kinds of grand-narrative approaches are insufficient for understanding the Prozac story. Prozac, like all technoscience, is too contradictory for sweeping claims to be of much help.

What the narratives of science and ethics have in common is that they are based on rather blunt distinctions: truth/myth for science and good/bad for ethics. Science asks: "Is Prozac science true, or is it a myth?" Ethics asks: "Is Prozac-induced happiness ethically good, or is it bad?" These narrative binaries are too coarse. With so many Prozac significations available, science can provide no grand truth of Prozac. What we have instead are many situated truths about Prozac. Similarly, bioethics can provide no single judgment of the good or the bad with regard to Prozac. In some ethical discourses, Prozac is a dawn of light for millions of depression sufferers; in others it is one of world's newest and most insidious and addictive of evils.

Cyborg theory helps us cut through these binaries. The undecidable situation of science and ethics does not mean that anything goes and certainly not that all technology should be embraced or rejected. Both technobliss and technophobia are held in tension in a cyborg reading. The undecidability of standard narratives does mean that we must develop an alternative discourse—besides the true or the false and the good or the bad—to scaffold and navigate questions of legitimacy in a posthuman world of cyborgs and cyborg technology.

But what alternatives for legitimizing technoscience discourse arise from Haraway's cyborg philosophy? In short, without recourse to universal truth or universal good, questions of legitimacy come down to local political questions of *consequences* and *inclusion*. What have been the particular consequences of Prozac? For whom? Who was included and empowered to create legitimate psychiatric knowledge regarding Prozac? Who was excluded, and why? Analyses of consequences and inclusions are midlevel discourses. They do not give sweeping or universal solutions; they only give temporary and situated ones. They result in messy and muddled conclusions because questions of consequences are diffuse and often go in contradictory directions. Questions of inclusion are always transient, as stakeholder groups are constantly emerging and disbanding.

Moving then from science and ethics to consequences and inclusions, let me first consider the question of consequences for Prozac. If I start at a broad discursive level, what might be called a cultural semiotic level, one major consequence of Prozac was to support a new psychiatry psychopharmacologic discourse of human pain and suffering that has deeply conservative political ramifications. The new biopsychiatry, as a way of talking about and organizing human pain, minimizes the psychological aspects of depression—personal longings, desires, and unfulfilled dreams—and it thoroughly erases its social aspects—injustice, oppression, lack of opportunity, lack of social resources, neglected infrastructures, and systematic prejudices. Not only that, but the new biopsychiatry mystifies and naturalizes the scientific (and pharmaceutical) contribution to the discourse on depression, leaving alternative opinions increasingly difficult to sustain. Biopsychiatry, like other scientific discourses (and this is perhaps its most insidious hegemonic effect), presents itself as a discourse from nowhere. No one claims to decide that depression should be organized primarily around neurophysiology; this is supposed to just be "the way it is." Alternative opinions become just that, "opinions," compared not to other opinions but to "facts."

As a deeply conservative discourse, biopsychiatry benefits the currently dominant groups. To state the case polemically, anyone unhappy with the status quo and the emerging New World Order, Inc. should shut up and take a pill. Of course, who is most unhappy, and who represents the highest percentage of depressed persons? Women, people of color, the poor, and other victims of societal biases (Ussher 1992; Stoppard 2000; Kleinman 1988; Mirowsky and Ross 2003). Who would stand to benefit the most from a change in the social order? The same folks. In the bioscience discourse of depression, however, the personal is not political; the personal is biological. If we plug human suffering, misery, and sadness into the calculus of bioscience, there is no need to make changes in the social order; instead, we need only to jump-start some neurotransmitters. There is no need to reduce social harassment, discrimination, gross inequities in opportunity, or corporate-media-induced status anxiety; instead, just let them have pills. There is no need for workers to take time off from the job for personal healing, reconsidering life choices, making life changes. There is no need to build an infrastructure to support those who are unable, for whatever reason, to find ways to support themselves. Instead, all people/machines need to do is to take a pill and get back to the New World Order of hyperactive consumption/production.

However, it must be added that it is tricky to polemically read consequences directly from a discourse. If discourse readings are done in a heavy-handed way, they leave out the possibility of negotiated and oppositional resistance to the dominant perspective (Hall 1980, 136). Rather than rest with a broad discussion of the discursive currents of Prozac and biopsychiatry, I must be more specific. I must articulate in greater detail who were the winners and who were the losers in the case of Prozac.

One of the most clear and least contradictory sites of Prozac effects is the pharmaceutical company Eli Lilly. It can be argued that, more than anyone else, Eli Lilly benefited from the advent of Prozac. In 1996 alone, Eli Lilly sold $2.3 billion worth of Prozac—and that was 32 percent of Eli Lilly's total sales (Eli Lilly and Company 1998). If that money had been spent on psychotherapy, it would have employed twenty-three thousand psychotherapists (at $100,000 gross income) to provide forty-six million psychotherapy hours during that year. Don't get me wrong. I'm not suggesting that psychotherapy is a simple good, any more than Prozac is a simple good. Psychotherapy, no different from biopsychiatric techno-science, is also intertwined in political forces that are barely articulated and critiqued within the psychotherapy discourse community. But one can at least say in favor of psychotherapy that, compared to biopsychiatry, psychotherapeutic psychiatry is not backed by a major bioscience industry.

Indeed, pharmaceutical companies are increasingly taking advantage of their size and capital to aggressively market their products. According to the *New York Times*'s business page, pharmaceutical companies are rapidly transforming themselves from "research-driven companies" to ones that operate "more like Procter & Gamble, the maker of Tide." For these drug companies, it is now the "marketing executives, not scientists, who are in charge" (Petersen 2000). To give an example of the effect of this change, IMS Health reports that

> pharmaceutical company promotional spending directed toward physicians and consumers in the U.S. reached $13.9 billion in 1999, an 11% increase over 1998. Total promotional spending includes physician detailing, sampling, and both consumer and physician advertising and promotion. Direct-to-consumer advertising, which accounts for 13% of audited promotional spending, totaled $1.8 billion, up 40% from the previous year. (IMS Health 2000)

Eli Lilly's Prozac has been consistently near the top in promotional spending.

My point is not to get into a detailed comparison of the relative effects and marketing strategies of psychotherapeutic and pharmacologic psychiatry. Instead, it is to show through the comparison with alternative treatment options like psychotherapy that, whatever other effects Prozac has had, it has produced an enormous benefit for Eli Lilly. The money spent on Prozac was money not spent on other options, and the profit to Eli Lilly for their promotional efforts was huge. In 1996 alone, Eli Lilly made $1.5 billion in profit (Eli Lilly and Company 1998). With this kind of bottom-line success, unless we are to get into the slings and arrows of wealth, there seems to be little need for further discussions of the benefits of Prozac for Eli Lilly.

From here, however, things get more complicated. Compared to the benefits for Eli Lilly, the further effects of Prozac become increasingly muddled and the vectors of effect much more contradictory. For example, what were the effects of Prozac for clinical psychiatrists? The answer turns out to be mixed. Clinical psychiatrists certainly benefited in many ways. Being, for the most part, members of dominant groups (upper-middle-class and often white, male, and heterosexual), clinical psychiatrists benefited from the general status quo that biopsychiatry supports. In the 1990s, they could charge around $60–$75 for a half-hour visit for prescribing Prozac. That was not bad money: $120 an hour, forty hours a week, fifty weeks a year, came to around $240,000 gross income per year. Not only that, but through their prescription privileges, they got a leg up on their guild rivals—psychologists and social workers. But the vectors for clinical psychiatrists were not necessarily all positive. Indeed, clinical psychiatrists may eventually suffer greatly from the Prozac/biopsychiatry phenomena. Now that psychiatrists are no longer known as having skills in psychotherapy, that service is rapidly going to their rivals. And as for the prescribing service they provide, that service too may eventually be taken over by others: such as primary-care clinicians, neurologists, psychologists, and nurse practitioners. Thus, clinical psychiatrists were not necessarily clear winners here, at least not in the long run.

Of course, psychiatrists are no longer (if they ever were) a single group, and during the age of Prozac clinical psychiatrists were rapidly becoming the group with the least voice among psychiatrists. As if it came from a textbook in colonial conquest, psychiatry has been divided into three dramatically unequal status groups. These may be articulated as "clinical," "research," and "administrative" psychiatrists. Out of these groups, research and administrative psychiatrists benefited the most from Prozac and biopsychiatry: research psychiatrists because of their access to pharmaceutical monies and academic power, and administrative psychiatrists because they used biopsychiatry to justify limiting other clinical psychiatric expenses, thus increasing profits for health care systems and enhancing their own positions within these systems. Consequently, among psychiatrists, clinicians (the group with the largest numbers but the least power) were most likely to lose out, and this pretty much seems to be the case.

But what about consumers? Technomedicine, or more precisely, technoscience capitalism in medicine (like capitalism generally), is complicated with regard to consumer benefit. The mantra of business seminars is "Win-Win." That phrase is supposed to mean that when a business wins, the customer wins as well, and the other way around. Therefore, by this logic, companies do not exploit consumers; companies only help consumers achieve their desires—otherwise a smart consumer would not buy the company's product. However, as Jean Baudrillard has so effectively pointed out in his "autopsy of homo economicus," the loophole of the Win-Win mantra is that (particularly in a postmodern consumer society) desire is not fixed, and businesses can use a variety of methods to stimulate desire (1988, 35). Consider cigarette companies, or auto companies, or soda companies, or computer software companies. Are the desires these companies create necessary? Can those desires be said in any logical way to rest "in the consumer"? Baudrillard points out the tremendous fluidity of consumer desire. He makes a compelling argument that it is better not to view needs as the stimulus of production, but to view production as the stimulus of needs. In Baudrillard's words, "*the system of needs is the product of the system of production*" (1988, 42, italics original; see also Galbraith 2000).

If Baudrillard is even partially correct, there can be no simple analysis of the effect of Prozac for consumers. How much do "Prozac needs" start with consumers, and how much are they stimulated by psychiatry and the pharmaceutical companies? This is an unanswerable question, as it is impossible to determine authentic individual needs outside of their cultural context. Thus, there is little theoretical (or political) advantage in celebrating consumer "euphoria." However, there is no more advantage in a grand critique of consumer "dupes." In spite of the generally conservative discourse of biopsychiatry, the clear advantage to the pharmaceutical industry and powerful psychiatrists, and the capacity of the psychiatric/pharmaceutical alliance to stimulate individual desires, there are many ways that Prozac, like other technoscience, can also empower consumers. For example, consider the situation of the abused woman who gets enough energy and hope through Prozac to stand up to or leave "her man." Or, at the larger political level, perhaps the next Simone de Beauvoir, Adrienne Rich, Kwame Nkrumah, or Angela Davis will be on Prozac. Perhaps without Prozac this individual would curl up in a depressive self-loathing rather than change the world.

Still, although consumers may benefit, they would be right to be wary of technomedicine. In the case of Prozac, it seems clear that, at the bottom line, Eli Lilly and the most powerful psychiatrists benefit as much if not more than consumers. At best, consumers can hope for a kind of trickle-down benefit. Consumer wariness is further warranted by the unequal power relations among the pharmaceutical companies, powerful psychiatrists, clinical psychiatrists, and consumers. Consumers are not powerless, but they are at the bottom of this power hierarchy. In a conflict between what is good for the consumer and what is good for the pharmaceutical companies or powerful psychiatrists, who do you think will usually win? Pharmaceutical companies and powerful psychiatrists are likely to put their interests first. This choice to privilege their own interests may be conscious and Machiavellian, but just as likely it may occur in the form of unconscious blind spots to other people's needs relative to their own. That seems to leave two positions for consumers (and, from my perspective, for clinical psychiatrists as well)—outright paranoia and general skepticism. There seems little room for blind trust.

One thing should begin to be clear in this very limited analysis of the consequences of Prozac. The picture is much more complicated and problematic than the biopsychiatry literature or the drug company advertisements would suggest. Eli Lilly's advertising slogan, "Neuroscience: Improving Lives, Restoring Hope," may well be true. But improving whose lives and restoring whose hope? One gets the sense that the most improved lives and the most restored hopes came to Lilly's CEO and its major stockholders. Thus, whatever Prozac may have been, it was not simple progress for everybody. And it certainly cannot claim to be a necessary or a universally true discourse on depression. Biopsychiatry does not have a divine right to the discourse on depression. To be a legitimate discourse of depression, Prozac and biopsychiatry cannot hide behind a curtain of science that effaces controversy and hypes only positive claims. Biopsychiatry must play fair with other possible discourses.

The Politics of Cyborgs

This brings me to the question of inclusion, or what I call the posthuman politics of cyborgs. Cyborg politics are politics of inclusion. If we follow Haraway and other theorists into the "politics of truth," it becomes clear that one of the most consistent effects of power on truth is the disqualification and prohibition of local and alternative forms of knowledge. As a result, dominant knowledge formations too often arise from dominant groups. As Sandra Harding has put it, "Women and men cannot understand or explain the world we live in or the real choices we have as long as the sciences describe and explain the world primarily from the perspectives of the lives of dominant groups" (1991, 307).

In today's sausage factory of knowledge production, that is exactly the situation we face. Dominant groups explain the world through their control of knowledge production. Subordinate groups are excluded, and as a result, subordinate knowledges are excluded as well. In liberal societies, these knowledge disqualifications are not achieved primarily through the legal authority of censorship. But as Foucault reminds us, these disqualifications are made by the "ensemble of rules according to which the true and the false are separated and specific effects of power are attached to the true" (1980, 132). As I discuss at length in chapter 3, knowledge/power works through the existence of a particular politico-economic regime of the production of truth. From this standpoint, the key task in confronting the politics of technoscience is not that of restoring the purity of scientific practice by criticizing its ideological contents nor, for that matter, attempting to emancipate truth from power. Rather, the task is to "detach the power of truth from the forms of hegemony (social, economic, and cultural) within which it operates at the present time" (Foucault 1980, 133).

Thus, a central task in a posthuman politics of Prozac is to challenge the hegemonic regime of bioscientific (and increasingly administrative and research) psychiatry and its pharmaceutical company supporters. Because there are diminishing opportunities for challenging biopsychiatry within the current psychiatric discourse (the reigning ensemble of rules separating the true and the false no longer permits it), the only remaining opportunity is a politics of activism. Models for this kind of activism exist already in medicine. The medical activisms I have in mind start from the perspective that medicine is, all too often, part of people's problems rather than part of their solutions. These are activisms that build on the strategies that midwives have used in their battle against organized ob-gyn physicians and hospitals, that La Leche League groups have used to help make breastfeeding a possible alternative, and that ACT UP (AIDS Coalition to Unleash Power) has used in its battle with institutionalized medicine over HIV treatment and research. Perhaps the best rallying cry for these activisms has come from the newly emerging disabilities movement: "Nothing about us without us" (Charlton 1998). This is a cry for inclusion in knowledge formation more than anything else. It rests on the experience that knowledge that excludes key stakeholders too often shifts toward the interests of those included over those excluded.[3]

In all of these activisms, it is not that medicine is simply wrong or bad.

It is more that medicine is too powerful, too hegemonic, too self-serving, and too unresponsive to alternative points of view. The medical activist groups (like feminism and other new social movements before them), in the face of medicine's political power, adopt a variety of strategies. They work to change people's consciousness. They build networks of opposition and support. They lobby for protective legislation. And in general, they provide a community of resistance to dominant forms of truth and a community of support for alternative knowledge structures.

In the case of medications like Prozac, this kind of "posthuman activism" would ideally have sources and coalitions both internal and external to psychiatry. Internal activism would involve lobbying dominant psychiatry to reduce its alignment with technoscience and with pharmaceutical companies. This kind of activist politics is a politics of alignment. It is about forming coalitions. Presently, psychiatry is too aligned with the pharmaceutical companies and the technoscience they produce and encourage. Twenty percent of the APA's budget comes from pharmaceutical companies, and pharmaceutical companies are major supporters of psychiatric research (Breggin 1991, chap. 15). These bioscience industry dollars, in spite of blanket claims of "unrestricted research support," profoundly affect the direction of psychiatric knowledge. Internal activism in psychiatry would loosen the alignment with the drug companies and increase psychiatry's alignments with patients, consumers, and clinicians. Rather than dominant psychiatrists creating knowledge as unofficial representatives of the drug companies—at conferences funded by drug money or presenting research funded by drug money—psychiatrists would attempt to get more consumer and clinical contributions to psychiatric knowledge. Psychiatry would try to create a knowledge base that includes a variety of points of view. Some of this knowledge would be informed by science, but it would also include knowledge informed by the humanities, interpretive social inquiry, and the arts.

New alliances in psychiatry would likely reduce rather than increase consensus in the field. In direct opposition to the more usual understanding of progress in science, I see this kind of increasing dissensus in the field as a positive rather than a negative. Consensus in posthuman politics should not be seen as a sign of advance so much as a sign of exclusion. Thus, the goal of psychiatry at the present moment should not be increased consensus but increased appreciation of diversity. Internal psychiatric politics must bring the struggle around biopsychiatry back home within psychiatry itself. The ideal way to make this work, as I discuss extensively in the last chapter, is for the American Psychiatric Association to become (much more than it is now) a forum for diverse opinions about mental suffering, rather than continue its attempts to create a single truth about mental illness and a single standard of care. Funding for research inquiry, according to this view, must not be decided by experts within scientific psychiatry alone. Research inquiry must be decided by a more democratic and inclusive process. The resulting APA would be made up of a patchwork of overlapping alliances and knowledges, not one knowledge formation based on a single authorized truth. In this situation, it would be best to speak in the plural and rename the APA the American Association of Psychiatries.

External activism to psychiatry has already begun. This activism takes the form of grassroots organizations that provide an alternative discourse to psychiatric treatments. One such group is the consumer/survivor movement, and another, more specific to Prozac, is Prozac survivors' groups. These groups have Web pages, local chapters, newsletters, conferences, protest rallies, and so forth, and they use them as a kind of cultural politics. Similar to the consciousness-raising functions of activist groups, they provide a source of critique of dominant power structures. They read technoscience psychiatry against the grain, deconstruct ideological hierarchies, satirize and poke fun at the dominant position, explore alternative possibilities, and in general form their identity in opposition to the "Other" of psychiatric science (Morrison 2003).

Both internal and external psychiatric activists must eventually increase their efforts to lobby Congress for protective legislation. As in regulating the cigarette industry, regulating biopsychiatry and the pharmaceutical industry will require many fronts of activity. On the legislative front, we need laws that reduce the capacity of drug companies to support (and advertise through) conferences and organizations in which they have a direct conflict of interest. In addition, legislation is needed that gives people better work benefits to deal with emotional problems—for example, more time to process a depression rather than being forced back to work as soon as possible. We need legislation that would allow nonbiomedical treatments the same insurance support that mainstream bioscience treatment is given. Legislation is needed that would improve mental health benefits generally—particularly benefits for psychotherapy—which have all but eroded over the same years as Prozac's rise to dominance. Finally, we need legislation that takes seriously the fact that social ills and community distress are huge factors in mental health and well-being.

In(con)clusion

I must admit that the political tasks I have presented here are more suggestive than programmatic. In its simplest form, what I am seeking boils down to the priority of democracy over science in psychiatric knowledge production. Prozac, like other kinds of technoscience, is not clearly oppressive or liberatory. It is a contradictory mixture of both—sometimes one more than another, but always both. This makes the problem not Prozac itself but the politics of representation surrounding the production and circulation of Prozac discourse. More people must be included in the decision-making process about the consequences of these kinds of medications. And we must ask much more forcefully: Who is getting to speak? Who is being silenced? How can knowledge production proceed on a more level playing field? How can more diverse groups get involved with the production and application of psychiatric knowledge?

These questions will take us beyond the usual forms of scientific and ethical analysis and regulation. If we wait until technoscience knowledge (like Prozac) is produced and then attempt to regulate its safe and ethical use, we wait too long—just as we cannot delete an e-mail after it has been sent. The challenge of technomedicine like Prozac is not only to insure its safe and ethical use but also to create a more level playing field for its knowledge production. This is the topic I turn to in chapter 8.

CHAPTER EIGHT

Postempiricism

Imagining a Successor
Science for Psychiatry

As I discuss in chapter 3, Michel Foucault's detailed philosophical inquiries into the discursive histories of psychiatry, medicine, the human sciences, criminal punishment, and sexuality repeatedly reveal a complex interweaving between historical knowledge formations and social power relations. For Foucault, these mangled interweavings of knowledge and power are so complex and so unavoidable that it becomes impossible to think of historical knowledge formations without also thinking of the power relations of their birth and propagation. Thus, Foucault's work has been highly instructive for overturning the Enlightenment illusion of "value-free" knowledge and for situating historical knowledges within specific power relations. Foucault opens the door to complex cultural studies readings of psychiatry that would not be possible within the current psychiatric discourse community.

In this chapter, I argue that Foucault's power/knowledge insights have value for psychiatry beyond his historical looks at discursive formations and the cultural studies readings he inspires. To use a metaphor from the video age, Foucault's insights should be "run forward"—ideally fast-forward—and used in organizing future knowledge-making structures in psychiatry. To articulate how this might be possible, I propose adding to Foucault's insights the work of recent feminist epistemologists and applying the combination toward future psychiatric knowledge production. Feminist epistemologists are essential in this task because, like

Foucault, they have used insights into the co-occurrence of power and knowledge to critique historical and current knowledge formations. But unlike Foucault, feminist epistemologists have gone past critique to construct alternative visions for future knowledge-making practices.

Similar to Foucault's work, feminist epistemologies overturn the notion of "value-free" science and the once-hallowed fact/value distinction on which it stood. Donna Haraway sums up this alternative perspective in a phrase: "Facts are theory laden, theories are value laden, and values are history [and politics] laden" (1981, 477). If psychiatry were to follow through on this reversal and destabilization of the fact/value distinction, future psychiatric research would have to be restructured. In the current context of psychiatry, the fact/value distinction—along with the fraternal distinctions of objective/subjective, truth/myth, science/pseudoscience, knowledge/conjecture, context of justification/ context of discovery—is the key starting point for knowledge inquiry. Psychiatric knowledge production tends to be divided into the separate domains of scientific knowledge production and bioethical knowledge regulation and oversight. Thus, in psychiatric research centers, we have "research committees" and "ethics committees," each composed of separate people and separate procedures. Scientific research committees determine the pursuit of knowledge (the facts), and medical ethics committees determine how that knowledge should be used (the values).

Of course, there are some "ethics of medical research" devoted to the proper values at issue between psychiatric researchers and their subjects. But for the most part, ethics and science are so divided during the stages of knowledge production that there is no systematic infrastructure available that allows us to ask and negotiate the following questions: What kinds of psychiatric knowledges are good to pursue, and for whom are they good to pursue? Which of the available methods of knowledge inquiry are best for psychiatry? And on what ethical or political grounds do we exclude possible contributors to psychiatric knowledge? Instead, we have an infrastructure that philosopher of science Philip Kitcher calls "internal elitism" (2001, 133). As Kitcher puts it, scientific research actually takes place as follows:

> The channeling of research effort is subject to pressures from a largely uninformed public, from a competitive interaction among technological enterprises that may represent only a tiny fraction of the population, and from scientists who are concerned to study

problems of very particular kinds or to use the instruments and forms of expertise that are at hand. (2001, 126)

Internal elitism means that scientific experts, coming from a narrow stratum of society, make all of these key value decisions among themselves and effectively decide the psychiatric knowledge agenda for everyone else. The situation is only getting worse in the context of multinational pharmaceutical and biotech corporations, directly or indirectly, funding much psychiatric research. As a result, bioethics can do little good because it enters the process of psychiatric knowledge production too late to make a sufficient impact. When bioethical value considerations are relegated to questions of knowledge *use,* rather than questions of knowledge *production,* it is like closing the barn door after the cows have run through—or, to update this metaphor for a posthuman age, it is like trying to undo electric shock treatment through the production of reverse seizures.

Running Foucault forward, recognizing that power/knowledge interminglings are inescapable in knowledge production, would begin to change this situation. Foucault's theory of power/knowledge implies that political and ethical choices are at play throughout the process of knowledge production (not just at the points of knowledge use). As a result, postpsychiatry must build an infrastructure that includes politics and equitable power relations in the process of psychiatric knowledge production. This turn from an exclusive focus on scientific content to an equal focus on the relations of scientific production is at the heart of feminist epistemology. Philosopher of science Joseph Rouse extends this turn to include more general "postepistemological" approaches to "knowledge, evidence, justification and objectivity" (2004, 361). When psychiatry takes this postepistemological turn, it will mean that the field of participants in psychiatric knowledge production must be greatly expanded. And it will mean that "peer review" will no longer be limited to a narrow scientific evaluation by a narrow band of scientific insiders. In other words, the postepistemological turn means that internal elitism must change and there must be more stakeholders involved.

Running Foucault forward, we must admit that, without such changes in the research infrastructure, the United States has a deeply problematic system of psychiatric knowledge production. No amount of ethical safeguards geared toward knowledge use will change this situation. Bioscience and bioethics programs must start addressing the issue of politics. If they do not, it will be time to set up "biopolitics coalitions" and "biopolitics centers" (to augment the minimal effects of current "bioethics centers") across the country and across the world to pick up where bioscience and bioethics are falling short. In the larger domain of the "life sciences," biopolitical action is already gaining much momentum in Europe and India in the crisis and controversy over genetically modified crops. Before psychiatry reaches its own crisis over the misuse and mistrust of science, psychiatric research-as-usual must change.

Introducing Democracy

The single most important rallying cry for a postepistemological research structure can be summed up in a sound bite: "Democracy in Psychiatry." Historically, the call for democracy has been one of the most powerful political imaginaries for social change. Of course it is true that, like other discourses, the discourse of democracy is open-ended and its meaning flexible. What it means and where it is applied are open to creative insight and collaborative struggle. But as democratic theorists Ernesto Laclau and Chantal Mouffe argue, for the most part the language of democracy has been a "fermenting agent" that has successfully motivated a variety of progressive politics, from the women's movement, to African American civil rights, to gay and lesbian liberation, to environmental activism (1985, 155). Going back further, this is the same democratic imaginary abolitionists cited to combat slavery, suffragettes used in their struggles for the vote, and anti-imperialist resistance fighters mobilized against their colonial rulers (Smith 1998, 9).

It seems that once democratic discourse gets started, the call for "democracy" functions as a rallying cry for collective action in ever-new domains—even those domains previously removed from democratic language. As Laclau and Mouffe put it:

> Egalitarian discourses and discourses on rights play a fundamental role in the reconstruction of collective identities. At the beginning of this process in the French Revolution, the public space of citizenship was the exclusive domain of equality, while in the private sphere no questioning took place of existing social inequalities. However, as de Tocqueville clearly understood, once human beings accept the legitimacy of the principle of equality in one sphere they will attempt to extend it to every other sphere. (1990, 128)